Radiographic Imaging & Exposure

Radiographic Imaging & Exposure

Second Edition

Terri L. Fauber, EdD, RT (R)(M)

Associate Professor and Chair
Department of Radiation Sciences
School of Allied Health Professions
Virgina Commonwealth University
Richmond, Virginia

with 235 illustrations

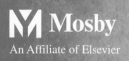 Mosby

An Affiliate of Elsevier

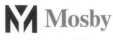

Mosby

An Affiliate of Elsevier

11830 Westline Industrial Drive
St. Louis, Missouri 63146

Previous edition copyrighted 2000

Library of Congress Cataloging-in-Publication Data

Fauber, Terri L.
    Radiographic imaging & exposure/Terri L. Fauber.–2nd ed.
        p.   cm.
    Includes index.
    ISBN 0-323-02557-9
    1. Radiography, Medical–Exposure.   2. Radiography, Medical–Image quality.
    I. Title: Radiographic imaging and exposure.   II. Title.
RC78.F33 2004
616.07′572–dc22

                            2003065158

Acquisitions Editor: Jeanne Wilke
Developmental Editor: Rebecca Swisher
Publishing Services Manager: Patricia Tannian
Project Manager: Sharon Corell
Design Manager: Bill Drone

Printed in the United States of America

Last digit is the print number: 9   8   7   6   5   4   3   2   1

CONTRIBUTORS

Terri L. Fauber, EdD, RT(R)(M)
Associate Professor and Chair
Department of Radiation Sciences
School of Allied Health Professions
Virginia Commonwealth University
Richmond, Virginia

Elizabeth Meixner, MEd, RT(R)(MR)(CT)
Assistant Chair
Department of Radiation Sciences
School of Allied Health Professions
Virginia Commonwealth University
Richmond, Virginia

Lori Nowicki Balmer, BGS, RT(R)(MR)
Clinical Coordinator, Radiography Program
Indiana University
South Bend, Indiana

Deanna Butcher, BSRT (R)
Program Director, Department of Radiology
    Education
St. Luke's College
Sioux City, Iowa

Anna M. Cox, BBA, RT(R)(M)
Instructor Radiology
Don Ana Branch Community College
Las Cruces, New Mexico

Eileen M. Doyle, MPA, RT(R)
Professor, Radiologic Technology
Monroe Community College
Rochester, New York

Charles Francis, MEd, RT(R)(QM)
Department Chair and Associate Professor
Idaho State University
Pocatello, Idaho

**Merryl N. Fulmer, BS,
RT(R)(M)(MR)(QM)(CT)**
Program Director
Abington Memorial Hospital
Abington, Pennsylvania

William F. Hennessy, MHS, RT(R)(M)(QM)
Assistant Professor, Clinical Coordinator
Quinnipiac University
Hamden, Connecticut

Beckey J. Miller, MS, RT(R)
Associate Professor
Horry-Georgetown Technical College
Conway, South Carolina

Kenneth A. Roszel, MS, RT(R)
Program Director, School of Radiologic
    Technology
Geisinger Health System
Danville, Pennsylvania

Alease Rousseau, BS, ARRT (R)
Program Director
Cleveland Community College
Shelby, North Carolina

Robert John Slothus, BS, MS, RT(R), ARRT
Director, Associate Professor
Pennsylvania College of Technology
Williamsport, Pennsylvania

Frances V. Williams, BS, RT
Director, Radiography Program
The Cooper Health System
Camden, New Jersey

Radiographic Imaging & Exposure provides a fundamental presentation of topics that are important for students to master to be competent radiographers. Radiographers will also benefit from the practical approach to the topics of imaging and exposure presented here. Historically in the United States, the most common reason for repeat radiographic studies has been improper exposure, and radiographic exposure remains one of the most difficult subjects for student radiographers to master. *Radiographic Imaging & Exposure* takes a unique and more effective approach to teaching the skills required by focusing on the practical fundamentals of imaging and exposure. With a topic such as radiographic imaging, it is impossible to depart from theoretic information entirely, and we do not want to. This book highlights the practical application of theoretic information to make it more immediately useful to students and practicing radiographers alike. Our ultimate goal is to provide the knowledge to problem solve effectively to consistently produce quality radiographic images in the clinical environment.

New to This Edition

As radiography moves to digital imaging, the knowledge and skills required of radiographers will change. This edition strives to integrate the basic concepts of digital imaging, where appropriate, throughout the chapters. The goal is to introduce this newer technology and compare and contrast it to film-screen radiography. An effort has been made to identify where the application of exposure principles of film-screen and digital imaging differ. Although digital imaging systems improve the consistency in producing quality radiographic images, the radiographer still ultimately controls the amount of radiation exposure to the patient. This responsibility cannot be overemphasized.

Chapter 4, Radiographic Quality, has been divided into two chapters, one on photographic properties and one on geometric properties. Chapter 11 in the first edition, Exposure Factor Modification, has been omitted and its content integrated in other chapters. Chapter 12 has been expanded to present other digital imaging systems in addition to computed radiography.

As in the first edition, a concerted effort was made to present the most important and relevant information on radiographic imaging and exposure. Radiation exposure and imaging will continue to be a complex subject, even in the digital age. As an educator who has struggled with the dilemma of how to best incorporate digital imaging within film-screen imaging courses, I strongly believe a solid foundation in the principles of radiation exposure will best prepare the student radiographer for digital imaging.

Content and Organization

Radiographic Imaging & Exposure begins with an intriguing discussion of Wilhelm Conrad Roentgen's discovery of x-rays in 1895 and the excitement it first caused among members of nineteenth-century society, who feared that private anatomy would be exposed for all to see! This introductory chapter moves into the realm of radiologic science with discussions of x-rays as energy and the unique characteristics of x-rays. Chapter 2 continues with a more detailed discussion of the x-ray beam, which is followed by chapters on radiographic image formation (Chapter 3), radiographic image quality: photographic properties (Chapter 4) and geometric properties (Chapter 5), scatter control (Chapter 6), and image receptors (Chapter 7). Chapter 8 is devoted to radiographic processing and includes important considerations about the darkroom environment, film handling, and quality control. Chapter 9 provides a thorough discussion of sensitometry, including important clinical considerations. Exposure factor selection is covered in Chapter 10 and automatic exposure control is covered in Chapter 11. Chapter 12 is devoted to digital imaging, including digital fluoroscopy. This final chapter explains the process of acquiring and displaying digital images and discusses the advantages and limitations of digital and conventional imaging processes.

Unique Features

Radiographic imaging and exposure is a complex topic, though a mastery of the fundamentals is necessary to become competent, whether you are a student or practicing radiographer. Three special features have been integrated within each chapter to facilitate the understanding and retention of the concepts under discussion and to underscore their applicability in a clinical setting. Each feature is distinguished by its own icon for easy recognition. The topic of radiographic imaging and exposure is replete with fundamental, important relationships, and they are emphasized in short, meaningful ways at every opportunity. Important Relationships summarize the relationships being discussed in the text, as each one occurs, for immediate summary and review. Radiographic imaging also has a strong quantitative component, and Mathematical Applications demonstrate the importance of mathematical formulas. This feature will help accustom you to the necessity of mastering mathematical formulas; because they are presented with clinical scenarios, they provide an immediate application and explanation. Practical Tips also provide immediate application of the concepts under discussion by showing how they are applied in clinical practice. The information in the chapters thus comes to life and encourages you to actively imagine how you would apply the knowledge you are learning in the classroom in a clinical setting. These special features also give the practicing radiographer quick visual access to fundamental information that they need every day.

Learning Aids

One of the primary goals of *Radiographic Imaging & Exposure* is to be a practical textbook that will prepare student radiographers for the responsibilities of radiographic imaging in a clinical setting. Every effort has been made to make the material easily accessible and understandable while remaining thorough. The writing style is straightforward and concise, and the textbook includes a number of features to aid in the mastery of its content. Relevant chapters include Film Critique sections that provide the opportunity to apply the science of imaging and exposure to the art of assessing actual radiographic image quality. Interpretations of the images in the Film Critique sections are collected in a final appendix for reference and discussion. All of the Important Relationships, Mathematical Applications, and Practical Tips are also collected in three separate appendixes for quick reference and review. These appendixes are organized by chapter and include page references to the appearance of each entry in the text. *Radiographic Imaging & Exposure* includes the traditional learning aids as well. Each chapter begins with a list of objectives and key terms and concludes with a set of multiple-choice review questions, which will help you evaluate whether you have achieved the chapter's objectives. An answer key is provided in the back of the book.

Teaching Aids

An instructor's manual contains material that is useful for both the practiced and novice educator. Each chapter features a set of learning objectives, different from the objectives listed in the text and designed specifically for the instructor. These objectives pull out and organize the key concepts of the chapters. The teaching strategies then provide ideas about how to help your students truly understand these concepts in addition to helping them master the stated chapter objectives. Usefulness is the key to the laboratory sections as well. The laboratory exercises accommodate different resources and instructor preferences by including both examples of predesigned experiments and additional recommended laboratory activities. We are also pleased to include more than 100 transparency masters of line drawings, boxes, and tables from the textbook. Finally, to further help you in your classroom instruction, we have provided a test bank of more than 200 questions, divided by chapter.

Related Multimedia

Wherever appropriate, we have included links in the instructor's manual to *Mosby's Radiographic Instructional Series:Radiographic Imaging*. This multimedia tool provides an additional resource to help in the mastery of the topics in *Radiographic Imaging & Exposure*. Mosby has developed multimedia presentations of basic physics, imaging, radiobiology, and radiation protection. These presentations are available in both slide/audiotape and CD-ROM formats.

Acknowledgments

It takes many dedicated people to create a textbook that will add to the body of knowledge about radiographic imaging and exposure. This textbook is a compilation of the creative works of its contributors, along with the support and encouragement from Mosby editors. Jeanne Wilke and Becky Swisher have demonstrated great patience and persistence in supporting this project throughout revision for the second edition. In addition, the many reviewers were instrumental in ensuring the book's focus and integrity. The vision Gary Watkins provided during the initial stages of the first edition was truly the driving force behind a practical textbook for radiographic imaging. Finally, radiography students' inquisitiveness and true desire for learning has inspired me to bridge the gap between radiographic imaging theory and practice.

We hope that this book will help you prepare for a successful career in radiography and that it will continue to serve you well in your clinical practice.

Terri L. Fauber

CONTENTS

Radiographic Imaging & Exposure

Radiation and Its Discovery

OBJECTIVES

1 Define all of the key terms in this chapter.
2 State all of the important relationships in this chapter.
3 Describe the events surrounding the discovery of x-rays.
4 Describe the dual nature of x-ray energy.
5 State the characteristics of electromagnetic radiation.
6 List the properties of x-rays.

KEY TERMS

fluorescence
electromagnetic radiation
wavelength

frequency
photon
quantum

X-rays were discovered in Europe in the late nineteenth century by German scientist Wilhelm Conrad Roentgen. Although Roentgen discovered x-rays by accident, he proceeded to study them so thoroughly that within a very short time, he had identified all of the properties of x-rays that are recognized today. Roentgen was less interested in the practical use of x-rays than in their characteristics as a form of energy. X-rays are classified as a specific type of energy termed *electromagnetic radiation*, but like all other types of electromagnetic energy, x-rays act both like waves and like particles.

Discovery

X-rays were discovered on November 8, 1895, by Dr. Wilhelm Conrad Roentgen (Figure 1-1), a German physicist and mathematician. Roentgen studied at the

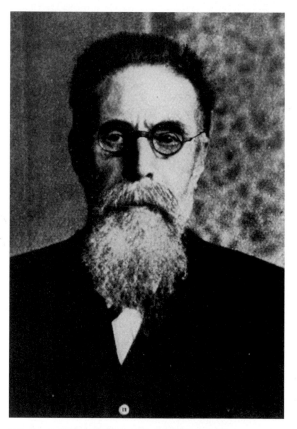

FIGURE 1-1 Dr. Wilhelm Conrad Roentgen.
From Glasser O: Wilhelm Conrad Roentgen and the early history of the roentgen rays, 1933.

Polytechnic Institute in Zurich. He was appointed to the faculty of the University of Würzburg and was their director of the Physical Institute at the time of his discovery. As a teacher and researcher, his academic interest dealt with the conduction of high-voltage electricity through low-vacuum tubes. A low-vacuum tube is simply a glass tube that has had some of the air evacuated from it. The specific type of tube that Roentgen was working with was called a *Crookes tube* (Figure 1-2).

Upon ending his workday on November 8, Roentgen prepared his research apparatus for the next experimental session to be conducted when he would return to his workplace. He darkened his laboratory to observe the electrical glow (cathode rays) that occurred when the tube was energized. This glow from the tube would indicate that the tube was receiving electricity and was ready for the next experiment. On this day, Roentgen covered his tube with black cardboard and again electrified the tube. By chance, he noticed a faint glow coming from some material located several feet from his electrified tube. The source was a piece of paper coated with barium platinocyanide. Not believing the cathode rays could reach that far from the tube, Roentgen repeated the experiment. Each time Roentgen energized his tube, he observed this glow coming from the barium platinocyanide paper. He understood that energy emanating from his tube was causing this paper to produce light, or fluoresce. **Fluorescence** refers to the instantaneous production of light resulting from the interaction of some type of energy (in this case x-rays) and some element or compound (in this case barium platinocyanide).

Roentgen was understandably excited about this apparent discovery, but he was also cautious not to make any early assumptions about what he had observed. Before sharing information about his discovery with colleagues, Roentgen spent time meticulously investigating the properties of this new type of energy. Of course, this new type of energy was not new at all. It had always existed and was likely produced

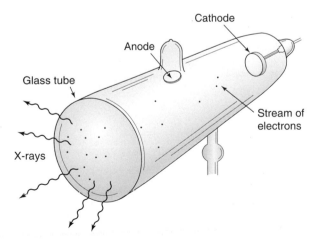

FIGURE 1-2 Crookes tube as used by Roentgen to discover x-rays.

by Roentgen and his contemporaries who were also involved in experiments with electricity and low-vacuum tubes. Knowing that others were doing similar research, Roentgen worked in earnest to determine just what this energy was.

Roentgen spent the next several weeks working feverishly in his laboratory to investigate as many properties of this energy as he could. He noticed that when he placed his hand between his energized tube and the barium platinocyanide–coated paper, he could see the bones of his hand glow on the paper with this fluoroscopic image moving as he moved his hand. Curious about this, he produced a static image of his wife Anna Bertha's hand using a 15-minute exposure. This became the world's first radiograph (Figure 1-3). Roentgen then gathered other materials and interposed them between his energized tube and the fluorescent paper. Some materials, such as wood, allowed this energy to pass through it and caused the paper to fluoresce. Some, such as platinum, did not.

In December 1895 Roentgen decided that his investigations of this energy were complete enough to inform his physicist colleagues of what he now believed to indeed be a discovery of a new form of energy. He called this energy x-rays with the

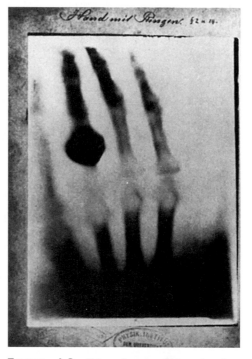

FIGURE 1-3 The first radiograph that demonstrates the bones of the hand of Roentgen's wife Anna Bertha with a ring on one finger.

From Glasser O: Wilhelm Conrad Roentgen and the early history of the roentgen rays, 1933.

x representing the mathematical symbol of the unknown. On December 28, 1895, Roentgen submitted a scholarly paper on his research activities to his local professional society, the Würzburg Physico-Medical Society. Written in his native German, his article was titled "On a new kind of rays," and it caused a buzz of excitement in the medical and scientific communities. Within a short time, an English translation of this article appeared in the journal *Nature*, dated January 23, 1896.

Roentgen viewed his discovery as an important one, but he also viewed it as one of primarily academic interest. His interest was in the x-ray itself as a form of energy, not in the possible practical uses of it. Others quickly began assembling their own x-ray–producing devices and exposed inanimate objects as well as tissue, both animal and human, both living and dead, to determine the range of use of these x-rays. Their efforts were driven largely by skepticism, not belief that x-rays could do what had been claimed. Skepticism eventually gave way to productive curiosity as investigations concentrated on ways of imaging the living human body for medical benefit.

As investigations into legitimate medical applications of the use of x-rays continued, the nonmedical and nonscientific communities began taking a different view of Roentgen's discovery. X-ray–proof underwear was offered as protection from these rays that were known to penetrate solid materials. A New Jersey legislator attempted to enact legislation that would ban the use of x-ray–producing devices in opera glasses. Both of these efforts were presumably aimed at protecting one from revealing their private anatomy to the unscrupulous users of x-rays. The public furor reached such a height that a London newspaper, the *Pall Mall Gazette*, offered the following editorial in 1896: "We are sick of Roentgen rays. Perhaps the best thing would be for all civilized nations to combine to burn all the Roentgen rays, to execute all the discoverers, and to corner all the equipment in the world and to whelm it in the middle of the ocean. Let the fish contemplate each other's bones if they like, but not us."

In a similar vein, but in a more creative fashion, another London newspaper, *Photography*, in 1896 offered the following:

> Roentgen Rays, Roentgen Rays?
> What is this craze?
> The town's ablaze
> With this new phase
> Of x-ray ways.
> I'm full of daze, shock and amaze,
> For nowadays
> I hear they'll gaze
> Through cloak and gown and even stays!
> The naughty, naughty Roentgen rays!

Fortunately, the scientific applications of x-rays continued to be investigated for the benefit of society, despite these public distractions. Roentgen's discovery was lauded as one of great significance to science and medicine, and Roentgen received the first Nobel prize presented for physics in 1901. The branch of medicine that was concerned with using x-rays was called *roentgenology*. A unit of radiation exposure was called the *roentgen*. X-rays were, for a time at least, called *roentgen rays*.

Excitement over this previously undiscovered type of energy was somewhat tempered by the realization in 1898 that x-rays could cause biologic damage. This was first noticed as a reddening and burning of the skin of those who were exposed to the large doses of x-rays required at that time. More serious effects, such as the growth of malignant tumors and the alteration of one's chromosomes, were attributed in later decades to x-ray exposure. Despite these disturbing findings, however, it was also realized that x-rays could be used safely. When radiation protection procedures are followed, which safeguard both radiographer and patient, x-rays assist medical diagnosis by imaging virtually every part of the human body.

X-RAYS as Energy

X-radiations, or x-rays, are a type of electromagnetic radiation. **Electromagnetic radiation** refers to radiation that has both electrical and magnetic properties. All radiations that are electromagnetic comprise a spectrum (Figure 1-4).

In the academic discipline of physics, energy can generally be described as behaving according to the wave concept of physics or the particle concept of physics. X-rays have a dual nature in that they behave both like waves and like particles.

Important Relationship

The Dual Nature of X-Ray Energy

X-rays act both like waves and like particles.

X-rays can be described as waves because they move in waves that have wavelength and frequency. If a sine wave were to be observed (Figure 1-5), it would be seen that **wavelength** represents the distance between two successive crests or troughs. Wavelength is represented by the Greek letter lambda (λ), and values are given in units of angstroms (Å). X-rays used in radiography range in wavelength from about 0.1 to 1.0 Å.

The sine wave (see Figure 1-5) also demonstrates that **frequency** represents the number of waves passing a given point per given unit of time. Frequency is represented by a lowercase *f* or by the Greek letter nu (ν), and values are given in units of Hertz (Hz). X-rays used in radiography range in frequency from about 3×10^{19} to 3×10^{18} Hz. Wavelength and frequency are inversely related. That is, as one increases, the other decreases.

THE ELECTROMAGNETIC SPECTRUM

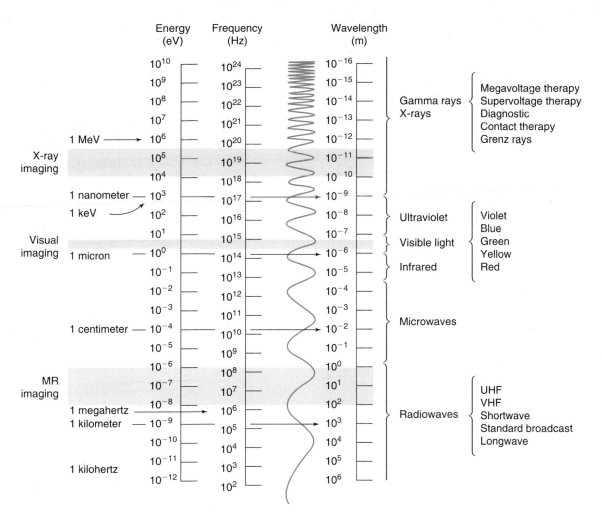

Figure 1-4 Electromagnetic spectrum. Radiowaves are the least energetic on the spectrum, and gamma rays are the most energetic.

Important Relationship

Wavelength and Frequency

Wavelength and frequency are inversely related. If one increases, the other decreases.

This relationship can be observed in Figure 1-6 and is demonstrated by the expression c = $\lambda\nu$ where *c* represents the speed of light. In this expression, if

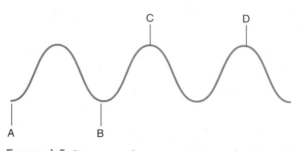

FIGURE 1-5 Sine wave demonstrating wavelength and frequency. One wavelength is equal to the distance between two successive troughs (points *A* to *B*) or the distance between two successive crests (points *C* to *D*).

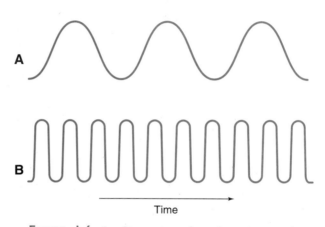

FIGURE 1-6 A, Sine wave that demonstrates long wavelength and low frequency. **B,** Sine wave that demonstrates short wavelength and high frequency. A comparison of sine waves **A** and **B** demonstrates the inverse relationship between wavelength and frequency.

wavelength increases, frequency must decrease because the speed of light is a constant velocity (3×10^8 m/s, or 186,000 miles/s). Conversely, if wavelength decreases, frequency must increase, again because the speed of light is constant.

X-rays also behave like particles and move as photons or quanta (plural). A **photon** or **quantum** (singular) is a small, discrete bundle of energy. For most applications in radiography, x-rays are referred to as *photons*. The energy of an individual photon is measured in units of electron volts (eV) and can be indicated by one of three expressions:

$$E = h\nu, \text{ or } E = hc/\lambda, \text{ or } E = 12.4/\lambda$$

where
E = Photon energy
h = Planck's constant (6.62×10^{-34} joules seconds)
c = The speed of light
ν = Frequency
λ = Wavelength.

Properties of X-Rays

X-rays are known to have several characteristics or properties. These characteristics are briefly explained here and presented in Box 1-1.

- *X-rays are invisible.* In addition to not being able to see x-rays, one can also not feel, smell, or hear them.
- *X-rays are electrically neutral.* They have neither a positive nor a negative charge; therefore they cannot be accelerated or made to change direction by a magnet or electrical field.
- *X-rays have no mass.* They create no resistance to being put into motion and cannot produce force.
- *X-rays travel at the speed of light in a vacuum.* They move at a constant velocity of 3×10^8 m/s or 186,000 miles/s in a vacuum.
- *X-rays cannot be optically focused.* Optical lenses have no ability in focusing or refracting x-ray photons.

Box 1-1 *Characteristics of X-Rays*

Are invisible.
Are electrically neutral.
Have no mass.
Travel at the speed of light in a vacuum.
Cannot be optically focused.
Form a polyenergetic or heterogeneous beam.
Can be produced in a range of energies.
Travel in straight lines.
Can cause some substances to fluoresce.
Cause chemical changes in radiographic and photographic film.
Can penetrate the human body.
Can be absorbed or scattered in the human body.
Can produce secondary radiation.
Can cause damage to living tissue.

- *X-rays form a polyenergetic or heterogeneous beam.* The x-ray beam that is used in diagnostic radiography is composed of photons that have many different energies. The maximum energy that a photon in any beam may have is expressed by the kilovoltage peak (kVp) that is set on the control panel of the radiographic unit by the radiographer.
- *X-rays can be produced in a range of energies.* These are useful for different purposes in diagnostic radiography. The medically useful diagnostic range of x-ray energies extends from 20 to 150 kVp.
- *X-rays travel in straight lines.* X-rays used in diagnostic radiography form a divergent beam in which each individual photon travels in a straight line.
- *X-rays can cause some substances to fluoresce.* When x-rays strike some substances, those substances produce light. These substances are used in diagnostic radiography, in intensifying screens, and in image intensifiers used in fluoroscopy.
- *X-rays cause chemical changes to occur in radiographic and photographic film.* X-rays are capable of causing images to appear on radiographic film and are capable of fogging photographic film.
- *X-rays can penetrate the human body.* X-rays have the ability to pass through the body, based on the energy of the x-rays and on the composition and thickness of the tissues being exposed.
- *X-rays can be absorbed or scattered by tissues in the human body.* Depending on the energy of an individual x-ray photon, that photon may be absorbed in the body or be made to scatter, moving in another direction.
- *X-rays can produce secondary radiation.* When x-rays are absorbed as a result of a specific type of interaction with matter, the photoelectric effect, a secondary or characteristic photon, will be produced.
- *X-rays can cause chemical and biologic damage to living tissue.* Through excitation and ionization of atoms comprising cells, damage to those cells can occur.

Since the publication of Roentgen's scientific paper, no other properties of x-rays have been discovered. However, the discussion of x-rays has expanded far beyond the early concerns about modesty or even danger. Today x-rays are accepted as an important diagnostic tool in medicine, and the radiographer is an important member of the health care team. The radiographic imaging professional is responsible for the care of the patient in the radiology department, as well as for the production and control of x-rays and the formation of the radiographic image. The balance of this book uncovers the intricate and fascinating details of the art and science of medical radiography.

Review Questions

1. In what year were x-rays discovered?
   A. 1892
   B. 1895
   C. 1898
   D. 1901

2. In what year were some of the biologically damaging effects of x-rays discovered?
   A. 1892
   B. 1895
   C. 1898
   D. 1901

3. X-rays were discovered in experiments dealing with electricity and
   A. ionization.
   B. magnetism.
   C. atomic structure.
   D. vacuum tubes.

4. X-rays were discovered when they caused a barium platinocyanide plate to
   A. fluoresce.
   B. phosphoresce.
   C. vibrate.
   D. burn and redden.

5. X-radiation is part of the _____ spectrum.
   A. radiation
   B. energy
   C. atomic
   D. electromagnetic

6. X-rays have a dual nature, which means that they behave like both
   A. atoms and molecules.
   B. photons and quanta.
   C. waves and particles.
   D. charged and uncharged particles.

7. The wavelength and frequency of x-rays are _____ related.
   A. directly
   B. inversely
   C. partially
   D. not

8. X-rays have a(n) _____ electrical charge.
   A. positive
   B. negative
   C. alternately positive and negative
   D. no charge

9. X-rays have
   A. no mass.
   B. the same mass as electrons.
   C. the same mass as protons.
   D. the same mass as neutrons.

10. The x-ray beam used in diagnostic radiography can be described as being
    A. homogeneous
    B. monoenergetic.
    C. polyenergetic.
    D. scattered.

CHAPTER 2

The X-Ray Beam

1 Define all of the key terms in this chapter.

2 State all of the important relationships in this chapter.

3 Describe construction of the x-ray tube.

4 State the function of each component of the x-ray tube.

5 Describe how x-rays are produced.

6 Explain the role of the primary exposure factors in determining the quality and quantity of x-rays.

7 Explain the line focus principle.

8 State how the anode heel effect can be used in radiography.

9 Calculate Heat Units.

10 State the purpose of an instantaneous load tube rating chart.

11 List the guidelines followed to extend the life of an x-ray tube.

KEY TERMS

cathode
filament
focusing cup
anode
target
stator
rotor
focal spot
leakage radiation
bremsstrahlung interactions
characteristic interactions
x-ray emission spectrum
filament current
thermionic emission
space charge
space charge effect

tube current
voltage ripple
line focus principle
actual focal spot size
effective focal spot size
anode heel effect
added filtration
inherent filtration
total filtration
half-value layer (HVL)
compensating filter
wedge filter
trough filter
heat unit (HU)
instantaneous load tube rating chart

The x-ray tube is the most important part of the x-ray machine because the tube is where the x-rays are actually produced. Radiographers must understand how the x-ray tube is constructed and how to operate it. The radiographer controls many of the actions that occur within the tube. Kilovoltage peak (kVp), milliamperage (mA), and exposure time are all factors that the radiographer selects to produce a quality image. The radiographer also needs to be aware of the amount of heat that is produced during x-ray production because excessive heat can damage the tube.

X-Ray Production

The production of x-rays requires a rapidly moving stream of electrons that are suddenly decelerated or stopped. The source of electrons is the cathode, or negative electrode. Electrons are stopped or decelerated by the anode, or positive electrode. Electrons move between the cathode and the anode because there is a difference in charge between the electrodes.

CATHODE

The **cathode** of an x-ray tube is a negatively charged electrode. It comprises a filament and a focusing cup. Figure 2-1 demonstrates a double-filament cathode surrounded by a focusing cup. The **filament** is a coiled tungsten wire that is the source of electrons during x-ray production.

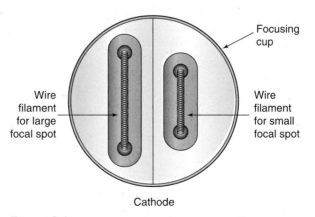

FIGURE 2-1 Most x-ray tubes use a small filament and a large filament, corresponding with a small focal spot size and a large focal spot size.

Important Relationship

The Filament.

The filament is the source of electrons during x-ray production.

Most x-ray tubes are referred to as *dual-focus tubes* because they use two filaments: a large filament and a small filament. Only one filament is energized at any one time during x-ray production. If the radiographer selects large focal spot when setting the control panel, the large filament is energized. If small focal spot is chosen, the small filament is energized.

The **focusing cup** is made of nickel and nearly surrounds the filament. It is open at one end to allow electrons to flow freely across the tube from cathode to anode. It has a negative charge, which keeps the cloud of electrons emitted from the filament from spreading apart. Its purpose is to focus the stream of electrons.

ANODE

The **anode** of an x-ray tube is a positively charged electrode. It consists of a target and, in rotating anode tubes, a stator and rotor. The **target** is a metal that abruptly decelerates and stops electrons in the tube current, thereby allowing the production of x-rays. The target can be either rotating or stationary. Rotating target tubes are more common than stationary ones. Rotating anodes are manufactured to rotate at a set speed ranging from 3000 to 10,000 revolutions per minute (RPM). Figure 2-2 demonstrates how a rotating and stationary anode differ in appearance.

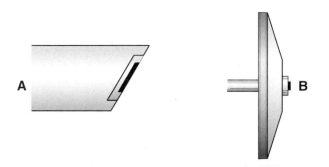

FIGURE 2-2 Side views of, **A,** a stationary anode and, **B,** a rotating anode.

The target is the part of the anode that is struck by the focused stream of electrons coming from the cathode. The target stops the electrons and thus creates the opportunity for the production of x-rays.

The target of rotating anode tubes is made of a tungsten and rhenium alloy. This layer, or track, is then embedded in a base of molybdenum and graphite (Figure 2-3). Tungsten generally makes up 90% of the composition of the rotating target, with rhenium making up the other 10%. The face of the anode is angled to help the x-ray photons exit the tube. Rotating targets generally have a target angle ranging from 6 to 20 degrees. Tungsten is used in both rotating and stationary targets because it has a high atomic number of 74 for efficient x-ray production and a high melting point of 3370° C. Most of the energy produced by an x-ray tube is heat, so melting of the target can sometimes become a problem, especially with high exposures.

Because tungsten has a high atomic number (74) and a high melting point (3370° C), it efficiently produces x-rays.

Almost all x-ray tube targets are made of tungsten. The only exception is the target of mammography x-ray machines. In mammography machines, molybdenum comprises 97% of the target. Like tungsten, molybdenum has a high melting point, but unlike tungsten, it produces a much lower-energy x-ray beam. An x-ray beam with lower energy is necessary for breast imaging because of the nature of breast tissue.

The **stator** is an electric motor that turns the rotor at very high speed during x-ray production. The **rotor** is rigidly connected to the target through the anode stem,

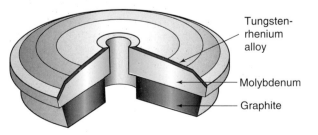

Tungsten-rhenium alloy

Molybdenum

Graphite

FIGURE 2-3 Typical construction of a rotating anode.

causing the target to rotate rapidly during x-ray production. High strength bearings in the rotor allow it to rotate smoothly at high speeds.

The purpose of the anode is also to dissipate heat away from the tube so that the tube is not damaged. Heat is transferred from the target through the anode stem to the rotor. The heat is then transferred to the glass envelope and to the insulating oil that surrounds the x-ray tube. Many tube assemblies also have a fan that blows air over the tube to help dissipate heat.

Important Relationship

Dissipating Heat

As heat is produced when the x-ray exposure is made, the rotating anode conducts the heat to the insulating oil that surrounds the x-ray tube.

Rotating anodes can withstand high heat loads. The ability to withstand high heat loads relates to the actual **focal spot,** which is the physical area of the target that is bombarded by electrons during x-ray production. With stationary targets the focal spot is a fixed area on the surface of the target. With rotating targets this area is represented by a focal track. Figure 2-4 shows the stationary anode's focal spot and the rotating anode with its focal track. The size of the focal spot is not altered with a

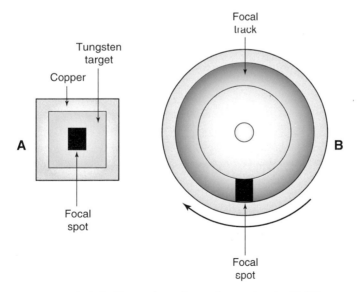

FIGURE 2-4 A, Front view of a stationary anode. **B,** The target area of the rotating anode turns during exposure, and there is an increased physical area—a focal track—that is exposed to electrons.

18   CHAPTER 2 *The X-Ray Beam*

rotating anode, but the actual physical area of the target bombarded by electrons is constantly changing, causing a greater area—a focal track—to be exposed to electrons. Because of the larger area of the target being bombarded during an exposure, the rotating anode is able to withstand higher heat loads produced by greater exposure factors. Rotating anode x-ray tubes are used in all applications in radiography, whereas stationary anode tubes are limited to studies of small anatomic structures such as the teeth.

> ### Important Relationship
>
> *Rotating Anodes*

Rotating anodes can withstand higher heat loads than stationary anodes because the rotation causes a greater physical area, or focal track, to be exposed to electrons.

X-RAY TUBE HOUSING

The components necessary for x-ray production are housed in a glass envelope. Figure 2-5 illustrates the structure of an x-ray tube, and Figure 2-6 shows the appearance of a typical x-ray tube. The glass envelope allows air to be evacuated completely from the x-ray tube, which allows the efficient flow of electrons from cathode to anode. The glass envelope serves two additional functions: it provides some insulation from electrical shock that may occur because the cathode and anode contain electrical charges, and it dissipates heat in the tube by conducting it to the insulating oil that surrounds the glass envelope. The purpose of insulating oil is to provide more insulation from electrical shock and to help dissipate heat away from the tube. All of these components are surrounded by a metal tube housing, except for

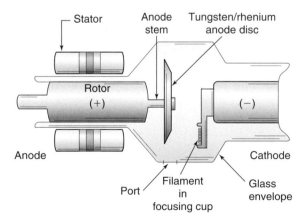

FIGURE 2-5 Structure of a typical x-ray tube, including the major operational parts.

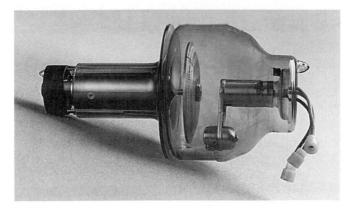

FIGURE 2-6 Typical x-ray tube as it appears before installation in a tube housing.

a port, or window, which allows the primary beam to exit the tube. It is the metal tube housing that the radiographer actually sees and handles when moving the x-ray tube. The tube housing is lined with lead to provide additional shielding from leakage radiation. **Leakage radiation** refers to any x-rays, other than the primary beam, that escape the tube housing. The tube housing is required to allow no more than 100 mR/hr of leakage radiation to escape when measured at 1 meter from the source while the tube operates at maximum output. Electrical current is supplied to the x-ray tube by means of two high-voltage cables that enter the top of the tube assembly.

RECENT INNOVATIONS

Two recent innovations in the design of modern diagnostic x-ray tubes have made them more efficient. One of these is the metal center section x-ray tube. A metal center section replaces the glass envelope in this region. In traditional x-ray tubes, tungsten that is evaporated from the filament during exposure deposits on the inside of the glass envelope, especially in the center of this envelope. This evaporation decreases the insulating ability of the tube and could lead to breakage of the glass, causing the tube to fail. Replacing this section of glass with metal prevents these problems and extends the tube life. The other innovation is the bonding of graphite to the back of the molybdenum disk used in rotating targets. Graphite has a high melting temperature and greatly assists in dissipating heat away from the tube.

Target Interactions

The electrons that move from the cathode to the anode travel extremely fast, approximately half the speed of light. The moving electrons, which have kinetic energy, strike the target and interact with the tungsten atoms in the anode to produce x-rays.

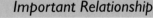

Important Relationship

The Production of X-Rays

As electrons strike the target, their kinetic energy is transferred to the tungsten atoms in the anode to produce x-rays.

These interactions occur within the top 0.5 mm of the anode surface. Two types of interactions produce x-ray photons: bremsstrahlung interactions and characteristic interactions.

Important Relationship

Interactions That Produce X-Ray Photons

Bremsstrahlung interactions and characteristic interactions both produce x-ray photons.

BREMSSTRAHLUNG INTERACTIONS

Bremsstrahlung is a German word meaning "braking" or "slowing down." **Bremsstrahlung interactions** occur when a projectile electron completely avoids the orbital electrons of the tungsten atom and travels very close to its nucleus. The very strong electrostatic force of the nucleus causes the electron to suddenly "slow down." As the electron loses energy, it suddenly changes its direction and the energy loss then reappears as an x-ray photon (Figure 2-7).

In the diagnostic energy range, most x-ray interactions are bremsstrahlung. The diagnostic energy range is 30 to 150 kVp. Below 70 kVp (with a tungsten target), 100% of the x-ray beam consists of bremsstrahlung interactions. Above 70 kVp, approximately 85% of the beam consists of bremsstrahlung interactions.

Important Relationship

Bremsstrahlung Interactions

Most x-ray interactions in the diagnostic energy range are bremsstrahlung.

CHARACTERISTIC INTERACTIONS

Characteristic interactions are produced when a projectile electron interacts with an electron from the inner (K) shell of the tungsten atom. The electron must have enough energy to eject the K-shell electron from its orbit. When the K-shell electron

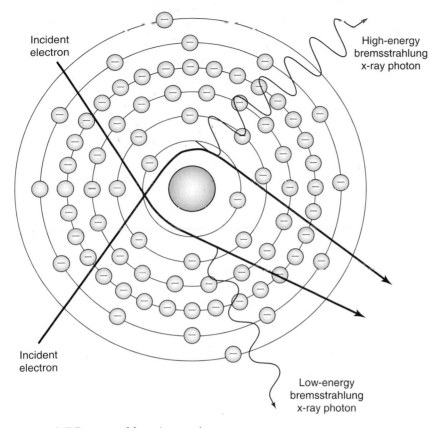

Incident electron

High-energy bremsstrahlung x-ray photon

Incident electron

Low-energy bremsstrahlung x-ray photon

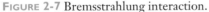

FIGURE 2-7 Bremsstrahlung interaction.

is ejected from its orbit, an outer-shell electron drops into the open position and thereby creates an energy difference. The energy difference is emitted as an x-ray photon (Figure 2-8). Electrons from the L-, M-, O-, and P-shells of the tungsten atom are also ejected from their orbits. However, the photons created from these interactions have very low energy and, depending on filtration, may not even reach the patient. K-characteristic x-rays have an average energy of approximately 69 keV; therefore they contribute significantly to the useful x-ray beam. Below 70 kVp (with a tungsten target), no characteristic x-rays are present in the beam. Above 70 kVp, approximately 15% of the beam consists of characteristic x-rays. X-rays produced through these interactions are termed *characteristic* x-rays because their energies are characteristic of the tungsten target element.

To summarize, when bremsstrahlung and characteristic interactions are compared, the majority of x-ray interactions produced in diagnostic radiology result from bremsstrahlung. There is no difference between a bremsstrahlung x-ray and a characteristic x-ray at the same energy level; they are simply produced by different processes.

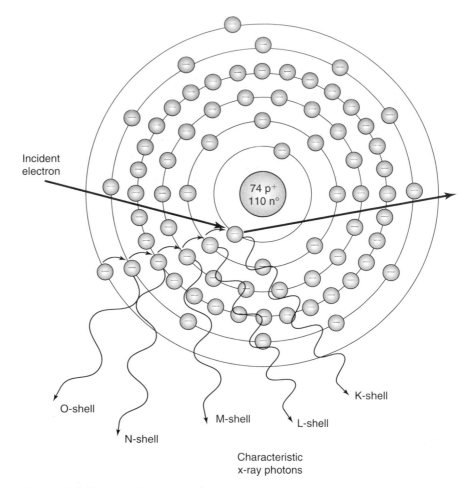

Incident electron

74 p$^+$
110 n°

O-shell

N-shell

M-shell

L-shell

K-shell

Characteristic
x-ray photons

FIGURE 2-8 Characteristic interaction.

X-Ray Emission Spectrum

X-ray energy is measured in kiloelectron-volts (keV) (1000 electron volts). The x-ray beam is polyenergenic and consists of a wide range of energies known as **x-ray emission spectrum.** The lowest energies are always approximately 15 to 20 keV, and the highest energies are always equal to the kVp set on the control panel. For example, an 80-kVp x-ray exposure technique produces x-ray energies ranging from a low of 15 keV to a high of 80 keV (Figure 2-9). The smallest number of x-rays occurs at the extreme low and high ends of the spectrum. The highest number of x-ray energies occurs between 30 and 40 keV for an 80-kVp exposure. The x-ray emission spectrum, or the range and intensity of x-rays emitted, changes with different exposure and kVp settings on the control panel.

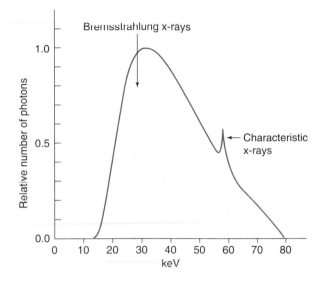

FIGURE 2-9 80-kVp x-ray emission spectrum from a tungsten target. Most x-rays occur between 30 and 40 keV.

X-Ray Exposure

A radiographic exposure is produced by a radiographer using two switches located on the x-ray unit's control panel. These are sometimes combined into a single switching device that has two levels of operation corresponding with the first and second switches. In either case the switches that are used to make an x-ray exposure are considered *deadman switches*. Deadman switches require positive pressure to be applied during the entire x-ray exposure process. If the radiographer lets off of either switch, releasing positive pressure, the exposure process is immediately terminated.

The first switch is usually called the *rotor*, or *prep button*, and the second switch is usually called the *exposure*, or *x-ray*, *button*. The activation of each switch by the radiographer produces specific reactions inside the x-ray tube. The rotor, or prep button, must be activated before the exposure, or x-ray, button is activated to properly produce an x-ray exposure.

Pushing the rotor, or prep button, causes an electric current to be induced across the filament in the cathode. This **filament current** is relatively low, approximately 3 to 5 amps, and operates at about 10 V. The amount of current flowing through the filament depends on the mA set at the control panel. The filament current heats the tungsten filament. This heating of the filament causes thermionic emission to occur. **Thermionic emission** refers to the boiling off of electrons from the filament.

Important Relationship

Thermionic Emission

When the tungsten filament gains enough heat *(therm)*, the outer-shell electrons *(ions)* of the filament atoms are boiled off, or *emitted*, from the filament.

The electrons liberated from the filament during thermionic emission form a cloud around the filament called the **space charge.** This term is descriptive because there is an actual negative charge from these electrons that exists in space around the filament. **Space charge effect** refers to the tendency of the space charge to not allow more electrons to be boiled off of the filament. The focusing cup, with its own negative charge, forces the electrons in the space charge to remain together.

By pushing the rotor, or prep button, the radiographer also activates the stator that drives the rotor and rotating target (Box 2-1). While thermionic emission is occurring and the space charge is forming, the stator starts to turn the anode, accelerating it to top speed in preparation for x-ray production. If an exposure could be made before the target is up to speed, the heat produced would be too great for the slowly rotating target, causing serious damage. The machine will not allow the exposure to occur until the target is up to full speed, even if the exposure switch is activated. Therefore the radiographer can press the rotor and exposure switches one after the other, and the machine will make the exposure as soon as it is ready, with no damage to the tube. It takes only a few seconds for the space charge to be produced and for the rotating target to reach its top speed (Figure 2-10).

When the radiographer pushes the exposure, or x-ray, button, the x-ray exposure begins (Box 2-2). The kVp level, which depends on the actual kVp value set on the

---

Box 2-1   *Preparing the Tube for Exposure*

When the rotor, or prep, button is pushed:

On the cathode side of the x-ray tube
1. Filament current heats up the filament.
2. This heat boils electrons off the filament (thermionic emission).
3. These electrons gather in a cloud around the filament (space charge).
4. The negatively charged focusing cup keeps the electron cloud focused together.
5. The number of electrons in the space charge is limited (space charge effect).

On the anode side of the x-ray tube
1. The rotating target begins to turn rapidly, quickly reaching top speed.

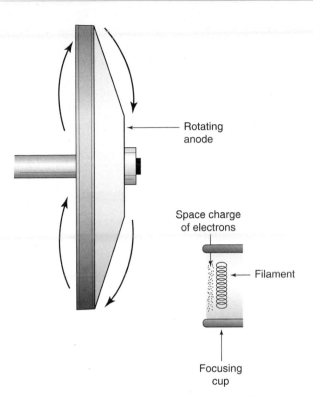

Rotating
anode

Space charge
of electrons

Filament

Focusing
cup

FIGURE 2-10 When the radiographer pushes the rotor, or prep button, a filament current is induced across the filament, causing electrons to be burned off and gather in a cloud around the filament. At the same time, the rotating anode begins to turn.

Box 2-2 *Making an X-Ray Exposure*

When the exposure, or x-ray, button is pushed:

On the cathode side of the x-ray tube
1. High negative charge strongly repels electrons.
2. These electrons stream away from the cathode and toward the anode (tube current).

On the anode side of the x-ray tube
1. High positive charge strongly attracts electrons in the tube current.
2. These electrons strike the anode.
3. X-rays and heat are produced.

control panel by the radiographer, is applied across the tube from cathode to anode. This creates potential difference and the cathode becomes highly negatively charged, strongly repelling the also negatively charged electrons. The anode becomes positively charged, strongly attracting the electrons. Electrons that comprised the space charge now flow quickly from cathode to anode in a current. **Tube current** refers to the flow of electrons from cathode to anode and is measured in units called milliamperes (mA). It is important to note that electrons flow in only one direction in the x-ray tube—from cathode to anode.

Important Relationship

Tube Current

Electrons flow in only one direction in the x-ray tube—from cathode to anode. This flow of electrons is called the *tube current* and is measured in milliamperes (mA).

As these electrons strike the anode target, they are converted to either x-rays or heat. In other words, an energy conversion occurs. The kinetic energy of the moving electrons is changed to electromagnetic energy (x-rays) and thermal energy (heat). Most of the electrons in the tube current (approximately 99%) are converted to heat, whereas only 1% (approximately) of these electrons are converted to x-rays. These events are illustrated in Figure 2-11.

Important Relationship

Energy Conversion in the X-Ray Tube

As electrons strike the anode target, approximately 99% of their kinetic energy is converted to heat, whereas only 1% (approximately) of their energy is converted to x-rays.

X-Ray Quality and Quantity

The radiographer initiates and controls the production of x-rays. Manipulating the prime exposure factors on the control panel (kVp, mA, and exposure time) allows both the quantity and quality of the x-ray beam to be altered. The quantity of the x-ray beam indicates the number of x-ray photons in the primary beam, and the quality of the x-ray beam indicates its penetrating power. Knowledge of the prime exposure factors and their effect on the production of x-rays will assist the radiographer in producing quality radiographs.

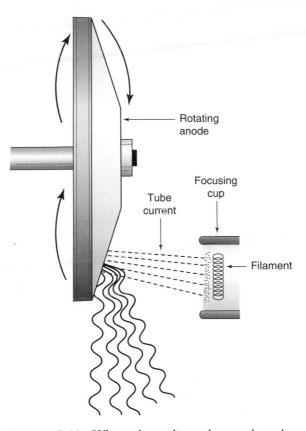

FIGURE 2-11 When the radiographer pushes the exposure, or x-ray button, a high voltage, or kilovoltage, is applied across the tube, making the cathode highly negative and the anode highly positive. Electrons are repelled from the cathode side and attracted to the anode side. The negatively charged focusing cup focuses the electrons into a stream, and they quickly cross the tube gap in a tube current. Electrons interacting with the target are converted into x-rays and heat.

KILOVOLTAGE

The kilovoltage (kVp) that is set by the radiographer and applied across the x-ray tube at the time the exposure is initiated determines the speed at which the electrons in the tube current move.

Important Relationship

Kilovoltage and the Speed of Electrons

The speed of the electrons traveling from the cathode to the anode increases as the kilovoltage applied across the x-ray tube increases.

A higher voltage results in greater repulsion of electrons from the cathode and greater attraction of electrons toward the anode. The speed at which the electrons in the tube current move determines the quality or energy of the x-rays that are produced. The higher the quality, or energy, of the x-ray photon, the greater the penetrability, or ease with which it moves through tissue. Whether one refers to the x-ray photons themselves or to the primary beam, *quality* and *energy* have the same meaning (Box 2-3).

Important Relationship

The Speed of Electrons and the Quality of the X-Rays

The speed of the electrons in the tube current determines the quality or energy of the x-rays that are produced. The quality or energy of the x-rays that are produced determines the penetrability of the primary beam.

Important Relationship

kVp and Beam Penetrability

As kVp increases, beam penetrability increases; as kVp decreases, beam penetrability decreases.

Box 2-3 *kVp and X-Ray Quality*

1. Higher kVp results in electrons that move faster in the tube current from cathode to anode.
2. The faster the electrons in the tube current move, the greater the quality of the x-rays produced.
3. The greater the quality of x-rays produced, the greater the penetrability of the primary beam.

In addition to kVp having an effect on the quality of x-ray photons produced, kVp has an effect on the quantity or number of x-ray photons produced. Increased kVp results in more x-rays being produced because increased kVp increases the efficiency of x-ray production.

To provide kilovoltage to the x-ray tube, providing sufficient potential difference to allow x-ray production, a generator is required to convert low voltage (volts) to high voltage (kilovolts). Three basic types of x-ray generators are available: single phase, three phase (capable of producing either 6 or 12 pulses per cycle), and high frequency. Each produces a different voltage waveform (Figure 2-12). These waveforms are a reflection of the consistency of the voltage supplied to the x-ray tube during an x-ray exposure. The term **voltage ripple** describes voltage waveforms in terms of how much the voltage varies during x-ray production. From Figure 2-12 it can be can be seen that for single-phase generation, voltage varies from the peak to a value of 0. Voltage ripple for single-phase generators is said to be 100% because there is total variation in the voltage wave-form, from peak voltage to 0 voltage. For three-phase generators, voltage ripple is 13% for 6-pulse, and 4% for 12-pulse. High-frequency generators produce a voltage ripple less than 1%. Voltage used in the x-ray tube is the most consistent with high-frequency generators. The more consistent the voltage applied to the x-ray tube throughout the exposure, the greater the quantity and quality of the x-ray beam.

MILLIAMPERAGE

A milliampere (mA) is the unit used to measure the tube current. Tube current measures the number of electrons flowing per unit time between the cathode and

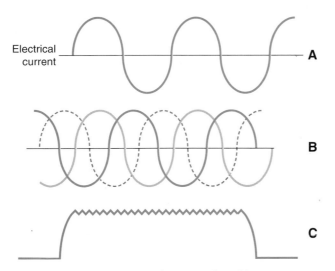

FIGURE 2-12 Voltage wave forms produced by various x-ray generators. **A,** Single Phase. **B,** Three Phase. **C,** High frequency.

anode. For example, at 100 mA there is a specific amount of current applied to the filament, causing a certain amount of thermionic emission. Based on the amount of thermionic emission, there is a space charge consisting of a certain number of electrons. 100 mA indicates the number of electrons (based on the space charge) flowing in the tube per second. Generally speaking, selecting the 200-mA station on the control panel causes twice as much thermionic emission, twice as big a space charge, and twice as many electrons to flow per second. The milliamperage that is set by the radiographer determines the number of electrons flowing in the tube and the quantity of x-rays produced (Box 2-4). The quantity of electrons in the tube current is directly proportional to the milliamperage. If the milliamperage increases, the quantity of electrons and the quantity of x-rays increases proportionally. If the milliamperage decreases, the quantity of electrons and the quantity of x-rays decreases by the same proportion. Milliamperage does not affect the quality, or energy, of the x-rays produced.

Important Relationship

Milliamperage, Tube Current, and X-Ray Quantity

The quantity of electrons in the tube current and quantity of x-rays produced are directly proportional to the milliamperage.

EXPOSURE TIME

Exposure time determines the length of time that the x-ray tube produces x-rays. The exposure time set by the radiographer can be expressed in seconds or milliseconds, either as a fraction or a decimal. This exposure time determines the length of time that the tube current is allowed to flow from cathode to anode. The longer the exposure time, the greater the quantity of electrons that will flow from the cathode to the anode and the greater the quantity of x-rays produced (Box 2-5). For example, if 400 mA at an exposure time of 0.25 second produces 5,000 x-rays, then an exposure time of 0.50 second at 400 mA will produce 10,000 x-rays. Changes in exposure time produce the same effect on the number of x-rays produced as do changes in milliamperage.

Box 2-4 *mA and X-Ray Quantity*

1. Higher mA results in more electrons that move in the tube current from cathode to anode.
2. The more electrons in the tube current, the more x-rays that will be produced.
3. The number of x-rays that are produced is directly proportional to the mA.

> ### Box 2-5 *Exposure Time and X-Ray Quantity*
>
> 1. Longer exposure time results in more electrons that move in the tube current from cathode to anode.
> 2. The more electrons in the tube current, the more x-rays produced.
> 3. The number of x-rays that are produced is directly proportional to the exposure time.

Important Relationship

Exposure Time, Tube Current, and X-Ray Quantity

The quantity of electrons that flows from cathode to anode and the quantity of x-rays produced are directly proportional to the exposure time.

MILLIAMPERAGE AND TIME

When milliamperage is multiplied by exposure time, the result is known as *mAs*, which the radiographer may be able to set at the control panel. Mathematically mAs is simply expressed as follows: $mA \times s = mAs$, where *s* represents exposure time in fractions of a second (as actual fractions or in decimal form) or in seconds.

Mathematical Application

Calculating mAs

$$mAs = mA \times seconds$$

Examples:

$$200 \text{ mA} \times .25 \text{ s} = 50 \text{ mAs}$$
$$500 \text{ mA} \times 2/5 \text{ s} = 200 \text{ mAs}$$
$$800 \text{ mA} \times 100 \text{ ms (milliseconds)} = 80 \text{ mAs}$$

The quantity of electrons that flows from cathode to anode is directly proportionate to mAs (Box 2-6). The quantity of x-ray photons produced is directly proportionate to the quantity of electrons that flows from cathode to anode. An increase or decrease in mA, exposure time, or mAs directly affects the quantity of x-rays produced; mAs has no effect on the quality of x-rays produced.

Box 2-6 *mAs and X-Ray Quantity*

1. Higher mAs results in more electrons that move in the tube current from cathode to anode.
2. The more electrons in the tube current, the more x-rays that will be produced.
3. The number of x-rays that are produced is directly proportionate to the mAs.

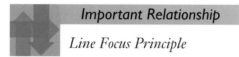

Important Relationship

The Quantity of Electrons, X-Rays, and mAs

The quantity of electrons flowing from the cathode to the anode and the quantity of x-rays produced are directly proportional to mAs.

Line Focus Principle

The **line focus principle** describes the relationship between the actual and effective focal spots in the x-ray tube.

Important Relationship

Line Focus Principle

The line focus principle describes the relationship between the actual focal spot, where the electrons in the tube current bombard the target, and the effective focal spot, that same area as seen from directly below the tube.

Actual focal spot size refers to the size of the area on the anode target that is exposed to electrons from the tube current. Actual focal spot size depends on the size of the filament producing the electron stream. **Effective focal spot size** refers to focal spot size as measured directly under the anode target. (Figure 2-13)

A tube's focal spot is an important factor because a large focal spot can withstand the heat produced by large exposures, whereas a small focal spot produces better image quality. The line focus principle demonstrates how, by angling the face of the anode, the actual focal spot can remain relatively large, while the effective focal spot is reduced in size. This allows for greater heat capacity while maintaining good image quality.

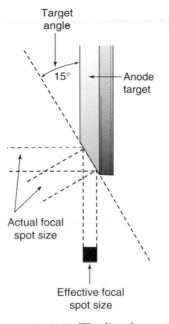

Target angle

15°

Anode target

Actual focal spot size

Effective focal spot size

FIGURE 2-13 The line focus principle addresses the relationship between the size of the actual focal spot (where the electrons actually bombard the target) and the effective focal spot (the same area as viewed and measured directly below the target).

When manufactured, every tube has a specific anode angle, typically ranging from 6 to 20 degrees. Based on the line focus principle, the amount of anode angle determines the size of the effective focal spot.

When an x-ray tube with a large target angle is used, a standard actual focal spot size is produced (based on the size of the filament) and a large effective focal spot size is produced. When an x-ray tube with a small target angle is used, the same size actual focal spot size is produced but a smaller effective focal spot results. The relationship among target angle, effective focal spot size, and actual focal spot size is illustrated in Figure 2-14.

Important Relationship

Anode Angle and Effective Focal Spot Size

Based on the line focus principle, the smaller the anode angle, the smaller the effective focal spot size.

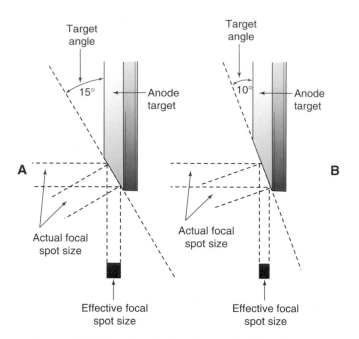

FIGURE 2-14 Based on the line focus principle, **A,** a large target angle will produce a large effective focal spot size and, **B,** a small target angle will produce a small effective focal spot size. Both actual focal spot sizes are the same, meaning that they can withstand the same heat loading.

Anode Heel Effect

A phenomenon known as the **anode heel effect** occurs because of the angle of the target. The heel effect describes how the x-ray beam has greater intensity (number of x-rays) on the cathode side of the tube, with the intensity diminishing toward the anode side (Figure 2-15).

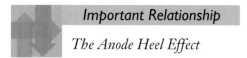

Important Relationship

The Anode Heel Effect

X-rays are more intense on the cathode side of the tube. The intensity of the x-rays decreases toward the anode side.

As x-rays are produced they leave the anode in all directions. The x-rays that are emitted toward the anode side of the tube are absorbed by the anode itself and are

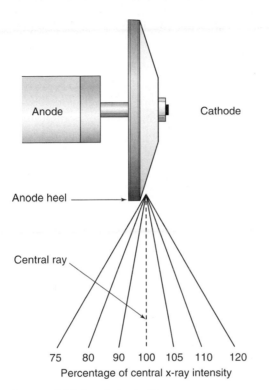

75 80 90 100 105 110 120

Percentage of central x-ray intensity

FIGURE 2-15 Anode heel effect.

therefore reduced in number in comparison to the photons that are emitted in the direction of the cathode. The difference in the intensities between the two ends can be as much as 45%. The heel effect can be used to advantage in radiography because the cathode end of the tube can be placed over the thicker body part, resulting in more even density on the radiograph.

Practical Tip

Using the anode heel effect

The anode heel effect can be used in imaging the thoracic spine, which has small vertebrae at the top and large vertebrae at the bottom. By placing the patient's head under the anode end of the tube, the more intense radiation will be directed toward the lower, larger portion of the spine and less intense radiation will expose the upper, smaller vertebrae.

Beam Filtration

The x-ray beam produced at the anode exits the tube housing to become the primary beam. This is the x-ray beam that eventually records the body part onto the image receptor. The x-rays that exit the tube are polyenergetic. They consist of low-, medium-, and high-energy photons. The low-energy photons are unable to penetrate the anatomic part and do not contribute to image formation. They contribute only to patient dose.

Important Relationship

Low-Energy Photons, Patient Dose, and Image Formation

Low-energy photons serve only to increase patient dose and do not contribute to image formation.

Reduction of the low-energy photons requires that filtration be added to the x-ray beam to attenuate or absorb these photons. **Added filtration** describes the filtration that is added to the port of the x-ray tube. Aluminum is the material primarily used for this purpose because it absorbs the low-energy photons while allowing the useful higher-energy photons to exit (Figure 2-16).

Various components within the x-ray tube assembly also contribute to the attenuation of low-energy x-rays. **Inherent filtration** refers to the filtration that is permanently in the path of the x-ray beam. Three components contribute to inherent filtration: (1) the glass envelope of the tube, (2) the oil that surrounds the tube, and (3) the mirror inside the collimator (beam restrictor located just below the x-ray tube) (Figure 2-16). **Total filtration** in the x-ray beam is the sum of the added filtration and the inherent filtration. The U.S. government sets standards for total filtration to ensure that patients receive minimum doses of radiation. The current guidelines state that x-ray tubes operating above 70 kVp must have a minimum total filtration of 2.5 mm of aluminum or its equivalent.

HALF-VALUE LAYER

Direct measurement of total filtration is usually not feasible, so an indirect process is used. **Half-value layer (HVL)**, the amount of filtration that reduces the intensity of the x-ray beam to one half its original value, is considered the best method for describing x-ray quality. Additionally, the HVL can be used as an indirect measure of the total filtration in the path of the x-ray beam. It is expressed in millimeters of aluminum (mm-Al). The U.S. government specifies the minimum value of HVL for all diagnostic x-ray tubes. If the HVL is at the appropriate level, the total filtration in the x-ray tube is adequate to protect patients from unnecessary radiation.

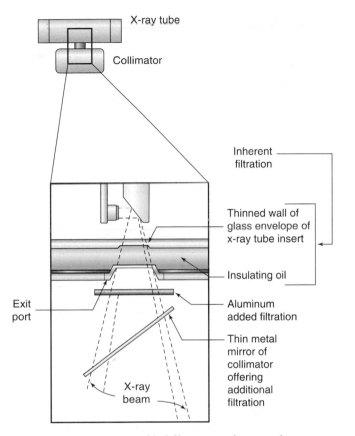

FIGURE 2-16 Aluminum added filtration is shown at the port, or window, of the x-ray tube. The inherent filtration of the glass envelope, the oil, and the collimator mirror are shown.

SPECIAL FILTERS

Special filters, called **compensating filters,** can be added to the primary beam to alter its intensity. These types of filters are used to image anatomic areas that are nonuniform in makeup, and assist in creating a radiographic image with more uniform density.

The most common type of compensating filter is a simple **wedge filter** (Figure 2-17, A). The thicker part of the wedge filter is lined up with the thinner portion of the anatomic part that is being imaged, allowing fewer x-ray photons to reach that end of the part. A wedge filter is commonly used for an anteroposterior (AP) projection of the femur, where the hip end is considerably larger than the knee end. A **trough filter** performs a function similar to the wedge filter; however, it is designed differently (Figure 2-17, B). The trough filter has a double wedge. A trough filter is commonly used for an AP projection of the thorax to compensate for the easily penetrated air-filled lungs.

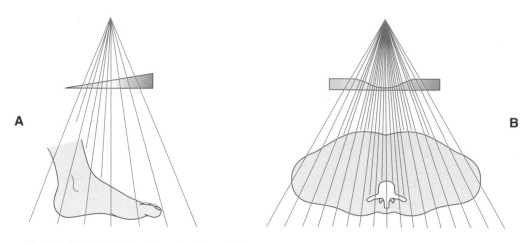

FIGURE 2-17 **A,** Wedge filter. **B,** Trough filter.

Heat Units

During x-ray production, most of the kinetic energy of the electrons is converted to heat. This heat can damage the x-ray tube and the anode target. The amount of heat produced from any given exposure is expressed by the **heat unit (HU).** The number of HUs produced depends on the type of x-ray generator being used and the exposure factors selected for a particular exposure, and can be expressed mathematically as:

$$HU = mA \times time \times KVp \times generator\ factor$$

The generator factor (Table 2.1) takes into account that the use of more consistent x-ray generators results in more heat.

TABLE 2-1   **THE GENERATOR FACTOR**

Generator Type	Factor
Single phase	1.00
Three phase 6 pulse	1.35
Three phase 12 pulse	1.41
High frequency	1.45

Calculating Heat Units

An exposure is made with a three phase, 12 pulse x-ray unit using 600 mA, and 0.05 seconds, 75 kVp. How many heat units are produced from this exposure?

$$HU = mA \times time \times kVp \times generator\ factor$$
$$HU = 600 \times 0.05 \times 75 \times 1.41$$
$$= 3172.5\ HU$$

Tube Rating Charts

Different models of x-ray tubes vary in their ability to withstand the heat produced by x-ray exposures. Manufacturers of x-ray tubes use instantaneous load tube rating charts, also called *single-exposure rating charts*, to describe the exposure limits of x-ray tubes. An **instantaneous load tube rating chart** is used to determine whether a particular exposure will be safe to make and to determine what limits on kVp, mA, and exposure time must be made to make a safe exposure. Violation of these limits as indicated by the tube rating chart will almost certainly result in permanent and irreparable damage to the x-ray tube. Figure 2-18 demonstrates a typical instantaneous load tube rating chart. For example, the maximum kVp that can be used with 700 mA and 0.3 second's exposure time is 90 kVp. The maximum mA that can be used with 105 kVp and 0.2 second's exposure time is 600 mA. The maximum exposure time that can be used with 85 kVp and 900 mA is 0.05 s. Whereas 130 kVp, 500 mA, and 0.1 s will produce a safe exposure, 130 kVp, 500 mA, and 0.2 s will not. Fortunately, manufacturers of today's x-ray units build their equipment so that tube-damaging exposures cannot be made. Generally, if an inappropriate technique is set, the radiographer will see a message such as "Technique Overload," or the machine may simply not expose after the rotor button is activated.

Extending X-Ray Tube Life

X-ray tubes are expensive devices that can fail because of radiographer error or carelessness. Not only do failed tubes result in an expense for purchasing a new tube, but there is also down time for a radiographic room when a failed tube is being replaced, decreasing productivity of that room. A few simple but important guidelines of x-ray tube operation should be adhered to consistently by the radiographer to extend tube life.

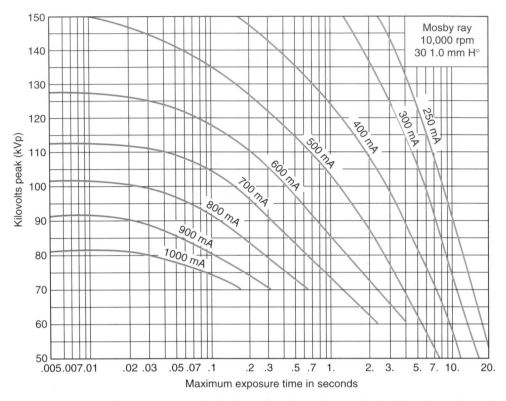

FIGURE 2-18 Typical instantaneous load tube rating chart that can be used to determine safe and unsafe exposures.

- Warm up the tube according to the manufacturer's specifications. It is always important to refer to the manufacturer's guidelines when warming up the tube, especially if it has not been energized for 2 hours or more.
- Avoid excessive heat unit generation. Observe and follow the limits that the tube's rating chart places on the various combinations of kVp, mA, and exposure time. Figure 2-19 shows anode targets that have been damaged as a result of excessive heat loading.
- Do not hold down the rotor button without making an exposure. Holding down the rotor button unnecessarily causes excessive wear on both the filament and the rotor.
- Use lower tube currents with longer exposure times when possible. This helps to minimize wear on the filament.
- Do not move the tube while it is energized. This movement can cause damage to the anode and anode stem as a result of torque, the force that acts to produce rotation.
- If the rotor makes noticeable noise, stop using the tube until it has been inspected by a qualified service person. Noises can be indicative of a potentially serious problem.

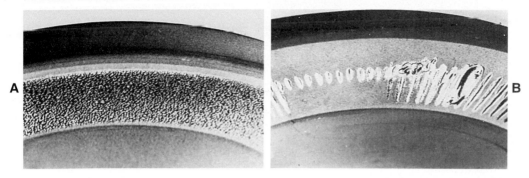

FIGURE 2-19 Two heat-damaged anode targets. **A,** Target shows pitting of the anode track caused by consistent overloading of exposure factors. **B,** Target shows melting of the focal track caused by failure of the rotor to rotate the anode. This failure usually results from heat damage of the rotor bearings from overloading the exposure factors.

Radiographers create diagnostic images by producing an x-ray beam that provides visualization of anatomic structures. The x-rays produced by the radiographer affect not only the quality of the image but also the life of the x-ray tube. Understanding the prime exposure factors and their effect on the x-ray beam and knowing what happens inside the x-ray tube are important considerations in radiography.

Review Questions

1. Which x-ray tube component serves as a source of electrons for x-ray production?
    A. Focusing cup
    B. Filament
    C. Stator
    D. Target

2. Electrons interact with the _____ to produce x-rays and heat.
    A. focusing cup
    B. filament
    C. stator
    D. target

3. The cloud of electrons that forms before x-ray production is referred to as
    A. thermionic emission.
    B. space charge.
    C. space charge effect.
    D. tube current.

4. The burning or boiling off of electrons at the cathode is referred to as
    A. thermionic emission.
    B. space charge.
    C. space charge effect.
    D. tube current.

5. Which primary exposure factor influences both the quantity and the quality of x-ray photons?
    A. mA
    B. mAs
    C. kVp
    D. Exposure time

6. The unit used to express tube current is
    A. mA
    B. mAs
    C. kVp
    D. s

7. What percentage of the kinetic energy is converted to heat when moving electrons strike the anode target?
   A. 1%
   B. 25%
   C. 59%
   D. 99%

8. The intensity of the x-ray beam is greater on the
   A. cathode side of the tube.
   B. anode side of the tube.
   C. short axis of the beam.
   D. long axis of the beam.

9. According to the line focus principle, as the target angle decreases, the
   A. actual focal spot size decreases.
   B. actual focal spot size increases.
   C. effective focal spot size decreases.
   D. effective focal spot size increases.

10. _____ will extend x-ray tube life.
    A. Selecting higher tube currents
    B. Using small focal spot when possible
    C. Producing exposures with a wide range of kVp values
    D. Warming up the tube after 2 hours of nonuse

Radiographic Image Formation

OBJECTIVES

1 Define all of the key terms in this chapter.

2 State all of the important relationships in this chapter.

3 Describe the process of radiographic image formation.

4 Explain the process of beam attenuation.

5 Describe the x-ray interactions termed *photoelectric effect* and *Compton effect*.

6 Define the term *ionization*.

7 State the composition of exit radiation.

8 State the effect of scatter radiation on the radiographic image.

9 Explain the process of creating the various shades of radiographic densities.

10 Define fluoroscopy and describe the process of image intensification.

11 Differentiate among conventional and digital imaging.

KEY TERMS

image receptor
differential absorption
attenuation
absorption
photoelectron
ionization
photoelectric effect
scattering
Compton effect
Compton electron/secondary electron

transmission
exit radiation
fog
latent/invisible image
manifest/visible image
fluoroscopy
image intensification
input/output phosphor
photocathode
electrostatic focusing lenses

To produce a radiographic image, x-ray photons must pass through tissue and interact with an **image receptor** (a device that receives the radiation leaving the patient), such as a film-screen system. Both the quantity and quality of the primary x-ray beam affect its interaction within the various tissues that make up the anatomic part. In addition, the composition of the anatomic tissues affects the x-ray beam interaction. The absorption characteristics of the anatomic part are determined by its composition, such as thickness, atomic number, and compactness of the cellular structures. Finally, the radiation that exits the patient will do so in varying energies, causing different shades of gray on the image receptor after processing.

Differential Absorption

The process of image formation is a result of **differential absorption** of the x-ray beam as it interacts with the anatomic tissue. Differential absorption is a process whereby some of the x-ray beam is absorbed in the tissue and some passes through (transmits) the anatomic part. The term *differential* is used because varying anatomic parts do not *absorb* the primary beam to the same degree. Anatomic parts composed of bone will absorb more x-ray photons than parts filled with air. Differential absorption of the primary x-ray beam will create an image that structurally represents the anatomic area of interest (Figure 3-1).

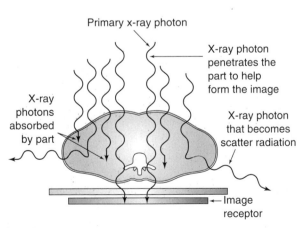

FIGURE 3-1 As the primary x-ray beam interacts with the anatomic part, photons will be absorbed, scattered, and transmitted. The differences in the absorption characteristics of the anatomic part create an image that structurally represents the anatomic part.

Differential Absorption and Image Formation

A radiographic image is created by passing an x-ray beam through the patient and interacting with an image receptor, such as a film-screen system. The variations in absorption and transmission of the exiting x-ray beam will structurally represent the anatomic area of interest.

Creating a radiographic image by differential absorption requires that several processes occur.

Beam Attenuation

As the primary x-ray beam passes through anatomic tissue, it will lose some of its energy. This reduction in the energy of the primary x-ray beam is known as **attenuation.** Beam attenuation occurs as a result of the photon interactions with the atomic structures that compose the tissues. Three distinct processes occur during beam attenuation: absorption, scattering, and photon transmission.

ABSORPTION

As the energy of the primary x-ray beam is deposited within the atoms composing the tissue, some x-ray photons will be completely absorbed. Complete **absorption** of the incoming x-ray photon occurs when it has enough energy to remove (eject) an inner-shell electron. The ejected electron is called a **photoelectron.** The ability to remove (eject) electrons, known as **ionization,** is one of the characteristics of x-rays. In the diagnostic range, this x-ray interaction with matter is known as the **photoelectric effect.**

With the photoelectric effect, the ionized atom has a vacancy, or electron hole, in its inner shell. An electron from an upper-level shell will drop down to fill the vacancy. Because of the difference in binding energies between the two electron shells, a secondary x-ray photon is emitted (Figure 3-2). This secondary x-ray photon is a form of scatter radiation and may exit the patient or interact with other tissue electrons.

X-Ray Photon Absorption

During attenuation of the x-ray beam, the photoelectric effect is responsible for total absorption of the incoming x-ray photon.

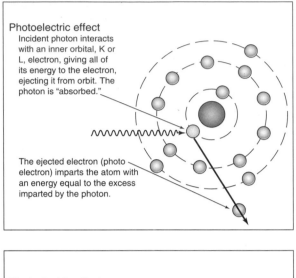

Photoelectric effect
Incident photon interacts with an inner orbital, K or L, electron, giving all of its energy to the electron, ejecting it from orbit. The photon is "absorbed."

The ejected electron (photo electron) imparts the atom with an energy equal to the excess imparted by the photon.

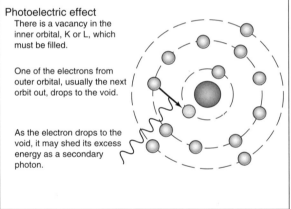

Photoelectric effect
There is a vacancy in the inner orbital, K or L, which must be filled.

One of the electrons from outer orbital, usually the next orbit out, drops to the void.

As the electron drops to the void, it may shed its excess energy as a secondary photon.

FIGURE 3-2 The photoelectric effect is responsible for total absorption of the incoming x-ray photon.

The probability of total photon absorption during the photoelectric effect is dependent on the energy of the incoming x-ray photon and the composition of the anatomic tissue. The energy of the incoming x-ray photon must be at least equal to the binding energy of the inner shell electron. After absorption of some of the x-ray photons, the overall energy of the primary beam will be decreased as it passes through the anatomic part.

SCATTERING

Some incoming photons are not absorbed, but instead they lose energy during interactions with the atoms comprising the tissue. This process is called **scattering** and results from the diagnostic x-ray interaction with matter, which is known as the **Compton effect.** The loss of energy of the incoming photon occurs when it ejects an outer-shell electron from the atom. The ejected electron is called a **Compton electron** or **secondary electron.** The remaining lower-energy x-ray photon changes direction and may leave the anatomic part to interact with the image receptor (Figure 3-3).

Important Relationship

X-Ray Beam Scattering

During attenuation of the x-ray beam, the incoming x-ray photon may lose energy and change direction as a result of the Compton effect.

If a scattered photon strikes the image receptor, it does not contribute any useful information about the anatomic area of interest. If scattered photons are absorbed within the anatomic tissue, they contribute to the radiation exposure to the patient. In addition, if the scattered photon leaves the patient and does not strike the image receptor, it could contribute to the radiation exposure of anyone near the patient.

Compton interactions can occur within all diagnostic x-ray energies and are therefore an important interaction in radiography. The probability of a Compton interaction occurring is dependent on the energy of the incoming photon. It is not dependent on the composition of the anatomic tissue. A Compton interaction is just as likely to occur in soft tissue as in tissue composed of bone.

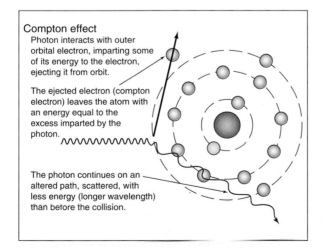

FIGURE 3-3 During the Compton effect, the incoming photon loses energy and changes its direction.

When comparing the likelihood of photoelectric interactions to Compton interactions, the percentage of photoelectric interactions generally decreases at higher kilovoltages within the diagnostic range, whereas the percentage of Compton interactions are likely to increase at higher kilovoltages within the diagnostic range.

Scattered and secondary radiations provide no useful information and must be controlled during radiographic imaging.

The preceding discussion focused on photon interactions that occur in radiography when using x-ray energies within the moderate range. Lower- and higher-energy x-rays result in other interactions (classic or coherent scattering, pair production, and photodisintegration) when the x-ray energies are beyond the moderate range used in radiography.

TRANSMISSION

If the incoming x-ray photon passes through the anatomic part without any interaction with the atomic structures, it is called **transmission** (Figure 3-4). At lower kilovotages, less x-ray transmission occurs, whereas at higher kilovoltages, more x-ray transmission occurs. The combination of absorption and transmission of the x-ray beam provides an image that structurally represents the anatomic part. Because scatter radiation is also a process that occurs during interaction of the x-ray beam and anatomic part, the quality of the image created is compromised if the scattered photon strikes the image receptor.

Practical Tip

X-Ray Interaction with Matter

When the diagnostic primary x-ray beam interacts with anatomic tissues, three processes occur during attenuation of the x-ray beam: absorption, scattering, and transmission.

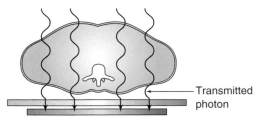

FIGURE 3-4 Some incoming x-ray photons will pass through the anatomic part without any interactions

EXIT RADIATION

When the attenuated x-ray beam leaves the patient, the remaining x-ray beam, referred to as **exit radiation,** is composed of both transmitted and scattered radiation (Figure 3-5). The varying amounts of transmitted and absorbed radiation (differential absorption) create an image that structurally represents the anatomic area of interest. Scatter exit radiation (Compton interactions) that reaches the image receptor does not provide any diagnostic information about the anatomic area. Scatter radiation creates unwanted density on the image called **fog.** Methods used to decrease the amount of scatter radiation reaching the image receptor are discussed in later chapters.

The areas within the anatomic tissue that absorb incoming x-ray photons (photoelectric effect) create the white or clear areas (low density) on the radiographic image. The incoming x-ray photons that are transmitted create the black areas (high density) on the radiographic image. Anatomic tissues that vary in absorption and transmission create a range of dark and light areas (shades of gray) (Figure 3-6).

Less than 5% of the primary x-ray beam interacting with the anatomic part actually reaches the image receptor and an even lower percentage is used to create the radiographic image. The exit radiation that interacts with an image receptor, such as a film-screen system, creates the **latent** or **invisible image.** This latent image will not be visible until the exposed film is developed and processed to produce the **manifest** or **visible image.**

Important Relationship

Image Densities

The range of image densities is created by the variation in x-ray absorption and transmission as the x-ray beam passes through anatomic tissues.

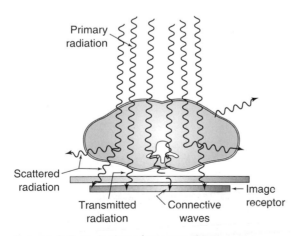

FIGURE 3-5 Radiation that exits the anatomic part comprises transmitted and scattered radiation.

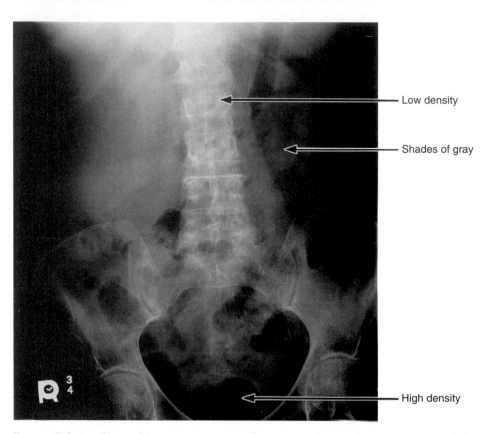

Low density

Shades of gray

High density

FIGURE 3-6 A radiographic image represents the various absorption characteristics of the anatomic part. An area of high density is where the x-ray beam was transmitted, and an area of low density is where the x-ray beam was absorbed. Anatomic tissues that vary in absorption and transmission create the shades of gray on the image.

Dynamic Imaging: Fluoroscopy

Fluoroscopy (Figure 3-7) allows imaging of the movement of internal structures. It differs from film-screen imaging by its use of a continuous beam of x-rays to create images of moving internal structures that can be viewed on a TV monitor. Internal structures, such as the vascular or gastrointestinal systems, can be visualized in their normal state of motion with the aid of special liquid substances (contrast media) that are injected or instilled.

Image intensification (Figure 3-8) is the process in which the exit radiation from the anatomic area of interest interacts with a light emitting material (**input phosphor**) for conversion to visible light. The light intensities are equal to the intensities of the exit radiation and are converted to electrons by a **photocathode** (photoemission). The electrons are focused by **electrostatic focusing lenses** and

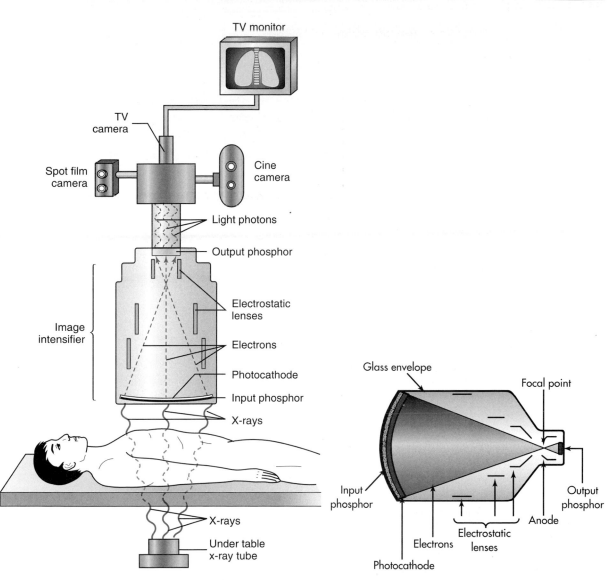

FIGURE 3-7 Fluoroscopic system used for dynamic imaging of internal structures.

FIGURE 3-8 Major components of an image intensifier. *(From Bushong SC: Radiologic Science for Technologists, 7th ed., St. Louis, Mosby, 2001.)*

accelerated toward an anode to strike the **output phosphor** and create a brighter image. The image light intensities from the output phosphor are converted to an electronic video signal and sent to a TV monitor for viewing.

Additional filming devices such as spot film or cine (movie film) can be attached to the fluoroscopic system to create permanent radiographic images of specific areas of interest.

Dynamic imaging of internal anatomic structures can be visualized with the use of an image intensifier. The exit radiation is absorbed by the input phosphor, converted to electrons, sent to the output phosphor, released as visible light, and then converted to an electronic video signal for transmission to the television monitor.

Digital Imaging

DIGITAL FLUOROSCOPY

The electronic video signal created from the output phosphor image light intensities during conventional fluoroscopy can be converted to digital (numeric) data and displayed on a high resolution TV monitor. Once the fluoroscopic image is digitized, a computer can manipulate the image in a variety of ways.

DIGITAL RADIOGRAPHY

Digital imaging can be accomplished by using a specialized image receptor that can produce a computerized radiographic image. Two types of digital radiographic systems are in use to today: computed radiography (CR) and direct readout digital radiography, commonly referred to as DR. Regardless of whether the imaging system is CR or DR, the computer can manipulate the radiographic image in a variety of ways after the image has been created digitally.

The process of differential absorption for image formation remains the same for digital imaging. The varying x-ray intensities exiting the anatomic area of interest form the latent image. In digital imaging the latent image is stored as digital data and must be processed by the computer for viewing.

Whether the radiographic image is created on film, a TV monitor, or a computer screen, the process of differential absorption for image formation remains the same. The varying x-ray intensities exiting the anatomic area of interest form the latent image.

Several important steps in creating a radiographic image have been discussed in this and the previous chapters. Further discussion of radiographic image quality, image receptors, control of scatter radiation, exposure technique selection, and problem solving are included in subsequent chapters.

Review Questions

1. The process whereby a radiographic image is created by passing an x-ray beam through anatomic tissue is known as
   A. attenuation.
   B. the photoelectric effect.
   C. the Compton effect.
   D. differential absorption.

2. Which of the following processes occur during beam attenuation: (1) absorption, (2) photon transmission, or (3) scattering?
   A. 1 and 2 only
   B. 1 and 3 only
   C. 2 and 3 only
   D. 1, 2, and 3

3. The ability of an x-ray photon to remove an atom's electron is a characteristic known as
   A. attenuation.
   B. scattering.
   C. ionization.
   D. absorption.

4. The x-ray interaction responsible for absorption is
   A. differential.
   B. photoelectric.
   C. attenuation.
   D. Compton.

5. The x-ray interaction responsible for scattering is
   A. differential.
   B. photoelectric.
   C. attenuation.
   D. Compton.

6. Exit radiation is composed of which of the following: (1) transmitted radiation, (2) absorbed radiation, or (3) scattered radiation?
   A. 1 and 2 only
   B. 1 and 3 only
   C. 2 and 3 only
   D. 1, 2, and 3

7. What interaction creates unwanted density known as fog?
   A. Compton
   B. transmitted
   C. photoelectric
   D. absorption

8. The low-density areas on a radiographic image are created by
   A. transmitted radiation.
   B. scattered radiation.
   C. absorbed radiation.
   D. primary radiation.

9. An anatomic part that transmits the incoming x-ray photon will create an area of _____ on the radiographic image.
   A. fog
   B. low density
   C. high density
   D. gray

10. Development and processing of an exposed film will result in a(n)
    A. manifest image.
    B. latent image.
    C. invisible image.
    D. inert image.

11. Imaging the movement of internal structures is known as
    A. attenuation
    B. photoemission
    C. electrostatic focusing
    D. fluoroscopy

12. What image intensifier component converts the visible light intensities from the input phosphor to electrons?
    A. thermionic emission
    B. photocathode
    C. anode
    D. output phosphor

CHAPTER 4

Radiographic Image Quality: Photographic Properties

1 Define all of the key terms in this chapter.
2 State all of the important relationships in this chapter.
3 Define the necessary components of radiographic image quality.
4 Differentiate between the photographic and geometric properties of a radiograph.
5 Differentiate among an optimal, diagnostic, and unacceptable radiograph.
6 Define *radiographic density* and discuss the controlling and influencing factors.
7 State how mAs and kVp can be used to adjust a density error.
8 Calculate changes in mAs and kVp to adjust radiographic density.

9 Define *radiographic contrast* and discuss the controlling and influencing factors.
10 Calculate changes in kVp to adjust radiographic contrast.
11 Explain the methods used to obtain a desired level of radiographic contrast.
12 Discuss the importance of both density and contrast in the visibility of recorded detail.
13 Identify exposure technique modifications for the following considerations:
Body habitus, pediatric patients, projections and positions, soft tissue, casts and splints, and pathology.

visibility of recorded detail (photographic properties)
sharpness of recorded detail (geometric properties)
radiographic density
15% rule
SID
inverse square law
density maintenance formula
OID
anode heel effect

reciprocity law
radiographic contrast
high contrast
short-scale contrast
low contrast
long-scale contrast
film (image receptor) contrast
subject contrast
contrast medium
body habitus

A primary responsibility of the radiographer is to evaluate radiographic images to determine whether sufficient information exists for a diagnosis. Evaluating radiographic quality requires the radiographer to assess the image for both its **visibility of recorded detail (photographic properties)** and its **sharpness of recorded detail (geometric properties).** Radiographic quality is the combination of both the visibility and the sharpness of recorded detail (discussed in Chapter 5). The radiographer must be knowledgeable about the factors that affect the photographic and geometric properties of a radiographic image to produce radiographs of optimal quality (Figure 4-1). The following discussion will focus on photographic properties of film-screen (conventional) imaging. Differences in the application of exposure factors with digital radiography will be presented at the end of this chapter.

Photographic Properties (Visibility)

Photographic properties (visibility factors) of recorded detail are determined by the extent to which the structural components of the anatomic area of interest can be seen on the recorded image. The radiographer views the entire image to determine whether the recorded detail is visualized sufficiently. When the radiographer determines that the visibility of recorded detail is maximized, the image is of optimal photographic quality. If the radiographer determines that the visibility of recorded detail is adequate or acceptable, the image is of diagnostic photographic quality. In the event that the radiographer determines the recorded detail is not adequately visualized, the image is unacceptable and the study must be repeated. At this point, the radiographer must determine the factors that should be adjusted to improve the visualization of the recorded detail. Visibility of the recorded detail is achieved by the proper balance of radiographic density and radiographic contrast.

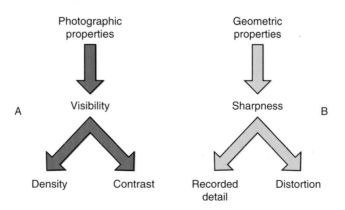

FIGURE 4-1 Factors affecting radiographic image quality. **A,** Photographic properties. **B,** Geometric properties.

Radiographic Density

Radiographic density is the amount of overall blackness produced on the image after processing. A radiograph must have sufficient density to visualize the anatomic structures of interest (Figure 4-2). A radiograph that is too light has insufficient density to visualize the structures of the anatomic part (Figure 4-3). Conversely, a radiograph that is too dark has excessive density, and the anatomic part cannot be well visualized (Figure 4-4). The radiographer must evaluate the overall density on the radiograph to determine whether it is sufficient to visualize the anatomic area of interest. He or she then decides whether the radiograph is optimal, diagnostic, or unacceptable. The ability to determine when a radiograph is unacceptable as a result of either insufficient or excessive density requires knowledge of the radiographic factors and clinical experience.

If a radiograph is deemed unacceptable, the radiographer must determine what factors contributed to the density error. Knowledge about the factors that affect the density on a radiograph is critical to developing effective problem-solving skills. Factors that directly affect density are identified as controlling factors, whereas influencing factors indirectly affect density (Box 4-1).

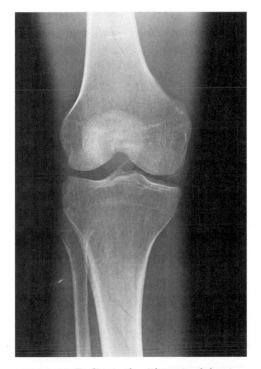

FIGURE 4-2 Radiograph with optimal density.

From Mosby's instructional radiographic series: radiographic imaging, St Louis, 1998, Mosby.

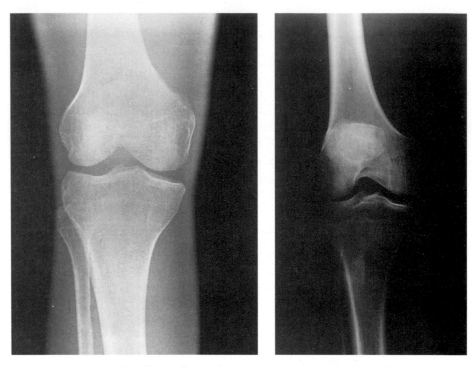

FIGURE 4-3 Radiograph with insufficient density.
From Mosby's instructional radiographic series: radiographic imaging, St Louis, 1998, Mosby.

FIGURE 4-4 Radiograph with excessive density.

Box 4-1 *Factors Affecting Density*

Controlling Factors	**Influencing Factors**
Milliamperage	Kilovoltage
Exposure time	Distance
	Grids
	Film-screen speed
	Collimation
	Anatomic part
	Anode heel effect
	Reciprocity law
	Generator output
	Filtration
	Film processing

CONTROLLING FACTORS

The quantity of radiation reaching the image receptor has a primary effect on the amount of radiographic density produced (Box 4-2).

Box 4-2 *Controlling Factors for Radiographic Density*

Milliamperage and exposure time control the quantity of radiation reaching the image receptor.

As discussed in Chapter 2, the product of milliamperage (mA) and exposure time (mAs) has a direct proportional relationship with the quantity of x-rays produced. When the quantity of x-rays is increased, the radiographic density also increases. Conversely, when the quantity of x-rays is decreased, the radiographic density decreases. Therefore radiographic density can be increased or decreased by adjusting the amount of radiation (mAs).

Important Relationship

mAs, Quantity of Radiation, and Radiographic Density

As the mAs is increased, the quantity of radiation is increased and radiographic density is increased. As the mAs is decreased, the amount of radiation is decreased and radiographic density is decreased.

Because mAs is the product of milliamperage and exposure time, increasing milliamperage or time has the same effect on density.

X Mathematical Application

Adjusting Milliamperage or Exposure Time

100 mA @ 0.10 s = 10 mAs. To increase the mAs to 20, you could use:

$$200 \text{ mA @ } 0.10 \text{ s} = 20 \text{ mAs}$$
$$100 \text{ mA @ } 0.20 \text{ s} = 20 \text{ mAs}$$

As demonstrated in the mathematical application, mAs can be doubled by doubling the milliamperage or doubling the exposure time. A change in either milliamperage or exposure time will proportionally change the mAs. To maintain the same mAs, the radiographer must increase the milliamperage and proportionally decrease the exposure time.

Important Relationship

Milliamperage and Exposure Time

Milliamperage and exposure time have an inverse relationship when maintaining the same mAs.

Mathematical Application

Adjusting Milliamperage and Exposure Time to maintain mAs

100 mA @ 100 ms (0.10 s) = 10 mAs. To maintain the mAs, you could use:

$$200 \text{ mA @ } 50 \text{ ms } (0.05 \text{ s}) = 10 \text{ mAs}$$
$$50 \text{ mA @ } 200 \text{ ms } (0.20 \text{ s}) = 10 \text{ mAs}$$

A change in mAs results in a direct change in density. For example, when the mAs is increased, density is increased; when the mAs is decreased, density is decreased (Figure 4-5).

When a radiograph is too light (insufficient density), a greater increase in mAs may be needed to correct the density, or the mAs may need to be decreased by more to correct a radiograph that has excessive density. This relationship between the quantity of radiation and density is discussed in more detail in Chapter 9.

The challenge for radiographers is to assess the level of density produced on a radiograph and to determine whether the density should be adjusted. When a radiograph is deemed unacceptable and the study must be repeated, the radiographer must decide how much of a change in mAs is needed to correct for the density error.

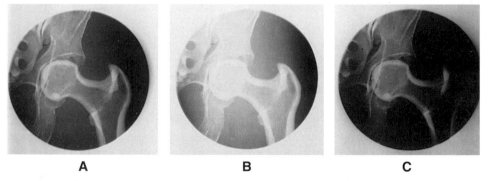

A   B   C

FIGURE 4-5 Changes in mAs have a direct effect on density. **A,** Original image. **B,** Decrease in density when the mAs is decreased by half. **C,** Increase in density when the mAs is doubled.

In general, for repeated radiographs that are necessary because of density errors, the mAs is adjusted by a factor of 2; therefore a minimum change involves doubling or halving the mAs. As mentioned previously, it may take more than doubling the mAs to correct for a density error. If the radiograph necessitates an adjustment greater than a factor of 2, the radiographer should multiply or divide the mAs by 4 (Figure 4-6).

Practical Tip

Repeating Radiographs Because of Density Errors

The minimum change needed to correct for a density error is determined by multiplying or dividing the mAs by 2. When a greater change in mAs is needed, the radiographer should multiply or divide by 4, 8, and so on.

Radiographs that have sufficient but not optimal density usually are not repeated. If a radiograph must be repeated because of another error, such as positioning, the radiographer may also use the opportunity to make an adjustment in density to produce a radiograph of optimal quality. Making a visible change in radiographic density requires that the minimum amount of change in mAs be approximately 30% (depending on equipment, somewhere between 25% and 35%). Radiographic studies generally are not repeated to make a slight visible change only. A radiographic study repeated because of insufficient or excessive density requires a change in mAs by a factor of at least 2.

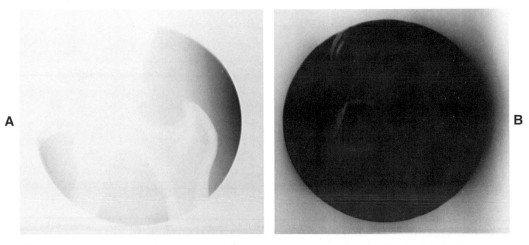

FIGURE 4-6 **A,** A greater increase in mAs, four times the original mAs, is needed. **B,** A greater decrease in mAs, one-fourth the original mAs, is needed.

INFLUENCING FACTORS

Although mAs is the controlling factor for radiographic density, other factors also affect density (see Box 4-1).

Kilovoltage

Kilovoltage peak (kVp) affects radiographic density because it alters the amount and penetrating ability of the x-ray beam. Increasing the penetration of the x-ray beam results in more radiation reaching the image receptor. As a result, more density is produced on the radiographic image (Figure 4-7).

Important Relationship

Kilovoltage and Radiographic Density

Increasing the kilovoltage peak increases the quantity of radiation reaching the image receptor and therefore increases radiographic density. Decreasing the kilovoltage peak decreases the quantity of radiation reaching the image receptor and therefore decreases radiographic density.

Kilovoltage has a direct relationship with density; however, the effect of kVp on density will not be equal throughout the range of kilovoltage (low, middle, and high).

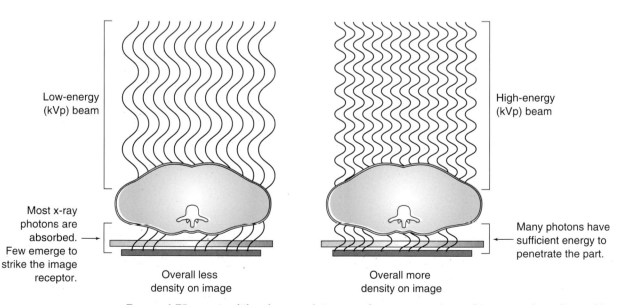

Low-energy (kVp) beam

High-energy (kVp) beam

Most x-ray photons are absorbed. Few emerge to strike the image receptor.

Many photons have sufficient energy to penetrate the part.

Overall less density on image

Overall more density on image

FIGURE 4-7 Increasing kilovoltage peak increases beam penetration and increases the radiographic density.

A greater change in kVp is needed when operating at a high kVp (greater than 90) compared with operating at a low kVp (less than 70) (Figure 4-8).

Kilovoltage affects not only the amount of density but also other aspects of the image; therefore kilovoltage is not the primary factor to manipulate for changes in radiographic density. However, it is sometimes necessary to manipulate the kilovoltage to maintain or adjust the density.

Maintaining or adjusting radiographic density can be accomplished with kilovoltage by using the **15% rule.** The 15% rule states that changing the kilovoltage peak by 15% will have the same effect on radiographic density as doubling the mAs, or reducing the mAs by 50%; for example, increasing the kilovoltage peak from 82 to 94 (15%) will have the same effect on density as increasing the mAs from 10 to 20.

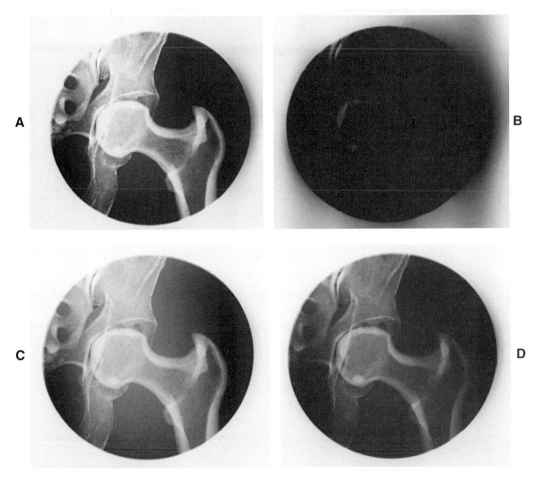

FIGURE 4-8 **A,** Produced at 50 kVp, and, **C,** produced at 90 kVp with the mAs adjusted to maintain radiographic density. **B,** A 10-kVp increase at 50 kVp will produce a greater change in density than, **D,** a 10-kVp increase at 90 kVp.

Practical Tip

Kilovoltage and the 15% Rule

A 15% increase in kilovoltage peak will have the same effect on radiographic density as doubling the mAs. A 15% decrease in kVp will have the same effect on radiographic density as decreasing the mAs by half.

Increasing the kVp by 15% increases the radiographic density, unless the mAs is decreased. Also, decreasing the kVp by 15% decreases the radiographic density, unless the mAs is increased. As mentioned earlier, the effects of changes in kVp are not uniform throughout the range of kVp. When low or high kilovoltages are used, the amount of change in kVp required to maintain the density may be greater or less than 15%.

X Mathematical Application

Using the 15% Rule

To increase density: Multiply the kVp by 1.15 (original kVp + 15%).

$$80 \text{ kVp} \times 1.15 = 92 \text{ kVp}$$

To decrease density: Multiply the kVp by 0.85 (original kVp − 15%).

$$80 \text{ kVp} \times 0.85 = 68 \text{ kVp}$$

To maintain density:

When increasing kVp by 15% (kVp × 1.15), divide the original mAs by 2.

$$80 \text{ kVp} \times 1.15 = 92 \text{ kVp and mAs/2}$$

When decreasing the kVp by 15% (kVp × 0.85), multiply the mAs by 2.

$$80 \text{ kVp} \times 0.85 = 68 \text{ kVp and mAs} \times 2$$

Distance

SID

The distance between the source of the radiation and the image receptor, source-to-image-receptor distance (**SID**) affects the amount of density produced on a radiograph. Because of the divergence of the x-ray beam, the intensity of the radiation will vary at different distances. This relationship between distance and x-ray beam intensity is best described by the **inverse square law,** which states that the intensity of the x-ray beam is inversely proportional to the square of the distance from the source. Because beam intensity varies as a function of the square of the distance, SID affects the quantity of radiation reaching the image receptor. As SID is increased, the x-ray intensity is spread over a larger area. This decreases the overall intensity of the x-ray beam reaching the image receptor. As SID increases, density decreases; as SID decreases, density increases(Figure 4-9). Because of the diverging properties of x-rays, changes in SID also affect other qualities of the image.

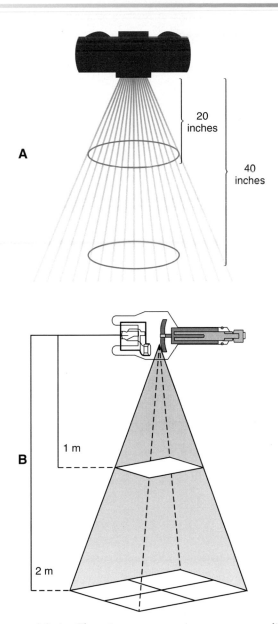

FIGURE 4-9 A, Changing source-to-image receptor distance (SID) and its effect on the divergence of the beam and, **B,** its effect on the intensity of the x-ray beam reaching the image receptor.

From Mosby's instructional radiographic series: radiographic imaging, St Louis, 1998, Mosby.

Important Relationship

SID and X-ray Beam Intensity

As SID increases, the x-ray beam intensity is spread over a larger area. This decreases the overall intensity of the x-ray beam reaching the image receptor.

Mathematical Application

Inverse Square Law Formula

$$\frac{I_1}{I_2} = \frac{(D_2)^2}{(D_1)^2}$$

The intensity of radiation at an SID of 40 inches is equal to 500 mR. What is the intensity of radiation when the distance is increased to 56 inches?

$$\frac{500\ \text{mR}}{X} = \frac{(56)^2}{(40)^2}$$

$$500\ \text{mR} \times 1600 = 3136X;\ \frac{800,000}{3136} = X\ ;\ 255.1\ \text{mR} = X$$

Important Relationship

SID and Radiographic Density

As SID increases, the radiographic density decreases as a result of the square of the distance. As SID decreases, the radiographic density increases as a result of the square of the distance.

Because increasing the SID decreases x-ray beam intensity and the density, the mAs must be increased accordingly to maintain density. When the SID is decreased, the density increases; therefore the mAs must be decreased accordingly to maintain density.

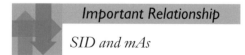

Important Relationship

SID and mAs

Increasing the SID requires that mAs be increased to maintain density, and decreasing the SID requires a decrease in mAs to maintain density.

Maintaining consistent densities when the SID is altered requires that the mAs be adjusted to compensate. The **density maintenance formula** (also known as *mAs/distance compensation formula*) provides a mathematical calculation for adjusting the mAs to change the SID.

 X *Mathematical Application*

Density Maintenance Formula

$$\frac{mAs_1}{mAs_2} = \frac{(SID_1)^2}{(SID_1)^2}$$

Optimal density is achieved at an SID of 40 inches using 25 mAs. The SID must be increased to 56 inches. What adjustment in mAs is needed to maintain radiographic density?

$$\frac{25}{mAs_2} = \frac{(40)^2}{(56)^2} \; ; \; 1600 \times = 78,400 \quad \frac{78,400}{1600} \; ; \; mAs_2 = 49$$

Standard distances are used in radiography to provide more consistency in radiographic quality. Most diagnostic radiography is performed at an SID of 40, 48, or 72 inches. Certain circumstances, such as trauma or mobile radiography, do not allow for standard distances to be used. In these circumstances the radiographer must determine the change needed in the mAs to obtain a radiograph with adequate density.

Practical Tip

Altering SID between 40 and 72 Inches

When a 72-inch SID cannot be used, adjusting the SID to 56 inches requires half the mAs. When a 40-inch SID cannot be used, adjusting the SID to 56 inches requires twice the mAs. This quick method of calculating mAs changes should produce sufficient density.

OID

When distance is created between the object radiographed and the image receptor, object-to-image receptor distance (**OID**), less density may result. As the exit radiation continues to diverge, less overall intensity of the x-ray beam will reach the image receptor. Although the amount of OID necessary to visibly affect image density has not been standardized, the radiographer should minimize the amount of OID whenever possible. OID has a greater effect on image contrast and sharpness.

Grids

A radiographic grid is a device that is placed between the patient and the image receptor to absorb scatter radiation exiting the patient. Limiting the amount of scatter radiation that reaches the image receptor improves the quality of the radiograph. Grids also absorb some of the transmitted radiation exiting the patient and therefore reduce the amount of density produced on a radiograph.

Important Relationship

Grids and Radiographic Density

Adding, removing, or changing a grid requires an adjustment in mAs to maintain radiographic density.

When grids are used, the mAs must be adjusted to maintain sufficient density. In addition, the more efficient a grid is in absorbing scatter, the greater the increase in mAs required to maintain the density. The grid conversion formula is a mathematical formula for adjusting the mAs for changes in the type of grid (Table 4-1).

When a grid is added, the radiographer must use the correct grid conversion factor to multiply by the mAs to compensate for the decreased density. When a grid is removed, the correct conversion grid factor must be divided into the mAs to compensate for the increased density. When the grid ratio is changed, the following formula should be used to adjust the density:

$$\frac{mAs_1}{mAs_2} = \frac{\text{Grid conversion factor}_1}{\text{Grid conversion factor}_2}$$

The new mAs will produce a density comparable to that of the original exposure technique.

TABLE 4-1   GRID CONVERSION CHART

Grid Ratios	Grid Conversion Factor
No Grid	1
5:1	2
6:1	3
8:1	4
12:1	5
16:1	6

Grids are primarily used to increase radiographic contrast and are discussed later in this chapter. The construction, conversion formula, and use of grids are discussed in more detail in Chapter 6.

X Mathematical Application

Adjusting mAs for changes in Grid

A quality radiograph is obtained using 2 mAs @ 70 kVp without using a grid. What new mAs is needed when adding a 12:1 grid to maintain radiographic density?

$$\frac{2 \text{ mAs}}{X} = \frac{1}{5}$$

$$2 \text{ mAs} \times 5 = 1 \text{ X}; 10 \text{ mAs} = X$$

Film-Screen Speed

The combination of the film and intensifying screen affects the image receptor's sensitivity to radiation exposure. The more sensitive the film-screen system is to radiation, the faster the speed. The speed of the film-screen system affects the amount of radiation required to produce a given amount of radiographic density. The greater the speed, the greater the density produced for a given exposure technique.

Important Relationship

Film-Screen System Speed and Radiographic Density

The greater the speed of the film-screen system, the greater the amount of density produced on the radiograph; the lower the speed of the film-screen system, the less density produced on the radiograph.

Because the film-screen system speed affects radiographic density, the mAs should be adjusted if the film-screen speed is changed. Increasing the film-screen system speed requires a decrease in the mAs to maintain radiographic density. A decrease in the film-screen system speed requires an increase in the mAs to maintain density.

Important Relationship

Film-Screen System Speed and mAs

Increasing the film-screen speed requires a decrease in the mAs to maintain density. Decreasing the film-screen speed requires an increase in the mAs to maintain density.

Film-screen systems are classified by their relative speed (RS) factor. Film-screen relative speeds range from 50 RS to as high as 800 RS. Extremity film-screen combinations usually have an RS of 100, and routine high-speed film-screen combinations have an RS of 400. The RS classification for film-screen systems provides a method whereby exposure techniques can be adjusted for changes in film-screen speed.

The relative film-screen speed conversion formula is a mathematical formula for adjusting the mAs for changes in the film-screen system speed.

$$\frac{mAs_1}{mAs_2} = \frac{RS_2}{RS_1}$$

The correct relative film-screen speed factors must be used to calculate the new mAs required to compensate for the change in density. The new mAs will produce a density comparable to that of the original exposure technique. Construction of films and intensifying screens and the screen conversion formula are discussed further in Chapter 7.

X Mathematical Application

Adjusting mAs for changes in Film-screen System Speed

A quality radiograph is obtained using 25 mAs @ 80 kVp and 100 speed film-screen system. What new mAs is used to maintain radiographic density when changing to a 400 speed film-screen system?

$$\frac{25 \text{ mAs}}{X} = \frac{400 \text{ spd.}}{100 \text{ spd.}}$$

$$25 \text{ mAs} \times 100 = 400X; \quad \frac{2500}{400} = 6.25 \text{ mAs} = X$$

Collimation

Any changes in the size of the x-ray field will alter the amount of tissue irradiated. A larger field size (decreasing collimation) increases the amount of tissue irradiated and increases the amount of scatter radiation reaching the image receptor, which in turn increases the amount of density on the radiograph. Conversely, a smaller field size (increasing collimation) reduces the amount of tissue irradiated and the amount of scatter radiation reaching the image receptor. This decrease reduces the amount of density on the radiograph.

Important Relationship

Collimation and Radiographic Density

Increasing collimation (smaller field size) decreases radiographic density; decreasing collimation (wider field size) increases radiographic density.

Anatomic Part

The thickness of the anatomic part being imaged affects the amount of x-ray beam attenuation that occurs. A thick part absorbs more radiation, whereas a thin part transmits more radiation.

Important Relationship

Part Thickness and Radiographic Density

A thick anatomic part decreases the radiographic density. A thin anatomic part increases radiographic density.

Maintaining density when imaging a thicker part requires the mAs to be increased accordingly. In addition, when a thinner anatomic part is being radiographed, the mAs must be decreased accordingly.

In general, for every change in part thickness of 4 cm, the radiographer should adjust the mAs by a factor of 2.

X Mathematical Application

Adjusting mAs for Changes in Part Thickness

An optimal radiograph was obtained using 40 mAs on an anatomic part that measured 18 cm. The same anatomic part is radiographed in another patient, and it measures 22 cm. What new mAs is needed to maintain density? Because the part thickness was increased by 4 cm, the original mAs is multiplied by 2, yielding 80 mAs.

Anode Heel Effect

As a result of the angle of the x-ray tube's anode, the intensity along the longitudinal axis of the primary x-ray beam varies; this variance is called the *anode heel effect*. The **anode heel effect** is a decrease in the primary x-ray beam intensity on the anode side of the tube, making the primary beam on the cathode side of the tube more intense in comparison. Under certain circumstances, this decrease in intensity at the anode end of the primary beam could affect the uniformity of densities produced and could be visible on the radiographic image.

The anode heel effect is more visible on radiographs that use a short SID and a large x-ray field size. When a short SID is used, the collimator (beam restricting device) must be opened further to achieve a particular projected field size. Opening the collimator more in the cathode-anode axis exposes the film to a wider variation in primary beam intensity. Likewise, the anode heel effect is less obvious on radiographs that use a long SID and a small field size. When a long SID is used, the collimator is opened less to achieve a particular projected field size. Opening the collimator less in the cathode-anode axis exposes the film to less variation in the primary beam intensity. The visibility of the anode heel effect on a radiographic image depends on the SID used, the x-ray beam field size, and the anatomic area of interest (Box 4-3).

Reciprocity Law

The **reciprocity law** states that the density produced on the radiograph will be equal for any combination of milliamperage and exposure time, as long as the product of mAs is equal. This law holds true for direct-exposure radiography (without intensifying screens). When intensifying screens are used to expose the film, reciprocity failure can occur when extreme exposure times are used. Exposure times of more than 10 s or less than 10 ms will not consistently produce the expected density for a given mAs. At these extreme exposure times, the intensifying screen light emission may not produce equivalent exposure of the film. The radiographer must use caution when operating at or below 10 ms. The density produced at this low exposure time may not be equal to the density produced at a higher exposure time and lower milliamperage combination. It is recommended that the radiographer select a reasonably low milliamperage to keep the exposure time to more than 10 ms so that sufficient density is produced.

Generator Output

Exposure techniques are developed in a radiographic room, and depend on the type of generator used. Generators with more efficient output, such as three-phase units, require lower technique settings to produce an image comparable to those of single-

---

Box 4-3 *Effective Use of the Anode Heel Effect*

To produce anteroposterior (AP) thoracic spine radiographs with relatively similar densities throughout all 12 vertebrae, the radiographer should position the patient so that the cathode side of the tube is over the inferior portion of the spine (abdomen) and the anode side of the tube is over the superior portion of the spine (chest). Likewise, for extremities, the cathode side of the tube should be positioned over the proximal end (thickest) of the extremity and the anode side of the tube should be positioned over the distal end (thinnest) of the extremity.

Placing the thickest part of the anatomic area under the cathode end of the x-ray beam will help decrease the visibility of the anode heel effect. Because the beam is more intense on the cathode side and less intense on the anode side, this technique generally produces a radiograph that is more uniform in density along the long axis of the image.

phase units. The radiographer must be aware of the generator output when using different types of equipment, especially when performing examinations in different departments. Refer to Chapter 2 for more discussion on generator output.

In addition, generator output variability can unexpectedly affect radiographic densities. X-ray generators must be calibrated periodically to ensure that they are producing consistent radiation output. Generator output variability is a quality control issue.

Tube Filtration

Small variations in the amount of tube filtration should not have any visible effect on the radiographic density. Variability of the x-ray tube filtration should be checked as a part of routine quality control checks on the radiographic equipment. X-ray tubes that have excessive or insufficient filtration may begin to affect the radiographic density. See Chapter 2 for a more thorough discussion of tube filtration.

Compensating Filters

Adding a compensating filter to the primary beam to produce more uniform radiographic density decreases the intensity of radiation interacting with the area of interest and image receptor. The use of compensating filters requires an increase in mAs to maintain the overall radiographic density without the compensating filter. The amount of increase in mAs is dependent on the thickness and type of compensating filter.

Film Processing

Processing of the film after exposure to radiation has a major effect on both the density and the contrast of the radiograph. Variability of the processor in temperature, chemistry, or film transport can adversely affect the radiographic density or contrast. A more thorough discussion of processing and its effect on exposed film can be found in Chapter 8.

Digital Imaging

The relationships among the exposure factors and their effect on the intensity of radiation also holds true for digital imaging. Changing the exposure factors of mAs, kVp, and SID will still alter the intensity of radiation reaching the image receptor as previously discussed.

The relationship between mAs and density is not the same for digital imaging as it is for film-screen imaging. Because a computer creates the image, the electronic data can be adjusted to correct for an error in the intensity of exposure reaching the image receptor. Although the computer can adjust for errors, the quality of the digital image may be adversely affected. In addition, radiographers may routinely use more exposure than required for the procedure, which in turn increases patient exposure.

It has been stated that exposure errors ± 50% can be adequately adjusted during digital image processing. Exposure errors beyond ± 50% can be adjusted, but the quality of the image may be sacrificed and the patient overexposed.

It is important for radiographers to select exposure factors that produce optimal quality images regardless of whether film-screen or digital image receptors are used. Selecting appropriate exposure factors ensures production of a quality image that provides the maximum amount of information needed for diagnosis with the least amount of exposure to the patient.

> ### Important Relationship
>
> *Exposure Factors and Digital Imaging*
>
> The relationship among the exposure factors of mAs, kVp and SID and their effect on the intensity of radiation reaching the image receptor holds true for digital imaging.

Radiographic Contrast

Radiographic contrast is a photographic factor that also affects the visibility of recorded detail. Contrast is the degree of difference between adjacent densities. The ability to distinguish between densities enables differences in anatomic tissues to be visualized. An image that has sufficient density but no differences in densities would appear as a homogeneous object (Figure 4-10). This appearance would indicate that the absorption characteristics of the object are equal. When the absorption characteristics of an object differ, the image presents with varying densities (Figure 4-11). In tissues where the absorption characteristics differ, visualization of recorded detail is optimal when contrast is maximized.

Radiographic contrast can be described as high or low. A radiograph with few densities but great differences among them is said to have **high contrast.** This is also described as **short-scale contrast** (Figure 4-12). A radiograph with a large number of densities but little differences among them is said to have **low contrast.** This is also described as **long-scale contrast** (Figure 4-13).

Radiographic contrast is the combined result of two categories: **film (image receptor) contrast** and **subject contrast** (Box 4-4). Film, or image receptor, contrast is a result of the inherent properties manufactured into the type of film and how it is radiographed (direct exposure or with intensifying screens), along with the processing conditions. Subject contrast is a result of the absorption characteristics of the anatomic tissue radiographed and the level of kilovoltage used.

Unlike density, contrast is a more complex photographic factor. Evaluating radiographic quality in terms of contrast is more subjective (it is affected by individual preferences). Furthermore, specifying the optimal level of radiographic contrast is difficult. The level of radiographic contrast desired in an image is determined by the composition of the anatomic tissue to be radiographed and the

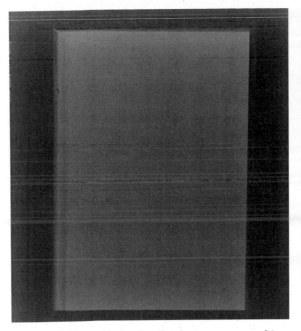

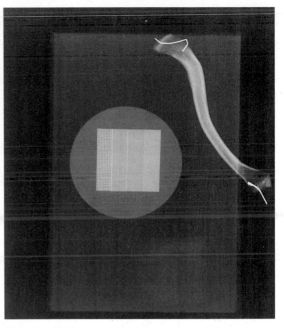

FIGURE 4-10 Radiograph of a homogeneous object having no differences in densities.

FIGURE 4-11 Object with different absorption characteristics produces an image with varying densities.

amount of information needed to visualize the tissue to make an accurate diagnosis. For example, the level of contrast desired in a chest radiograph is different from that required in a radiograph of an extremity. Also, the composition of the anatomic area varies greatly between the chest and an extremity.

The radiographer must evaluate the composition of the anatomic structure to be radiographed and determine the factors that must be manipulated to produce the desired level of radiographic contrast. Achieving the desired level of contrast maximizes the amount of information visible to make a diagnosis. As with density, the ability to produce the desired level of radiographic contrast depends on the radiographer's knowledge about the controlling and influencing factors and on his or her clinical experience.

Radiographic contrast can be evaluated best when the radiographic density is adequate to visualize the density differences. When density is either too light or too dark, radiographic contrast cannot be assessed adequately. Therefore the following discussion will focus on the factors that influence contrast, assuming radiographic density is adequate. This complex relationship between density and contrast is discussed in more detail in Chapter 9.

Factors that directly affect contrast are identified as controlling factors, whereas influencing factors indirectly affect contrast (Box 4-5).

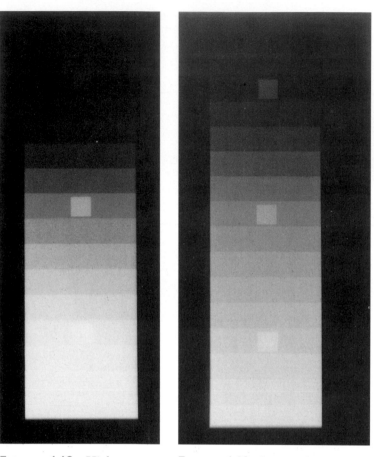

FIGURE 4-12 High-contrast (short-scale) image showing fewer gray tones and greater differences between individual densities.

FIGURE 4-13 Low-contrast (long-scale) image showing many gray tones and little difference between individual densities.

Box 4-4 *Factors in Radiographic Contrast*

Subject Contrast	Film (Image Receptor) Contrast
Kilovoltage	Film type
Tissue composition	Direct exposure or intensifying screens
Contrast medium	Processing conditions

Box 4-5 *Contrast*

Controlling Factor	**Influencing Factors**
Kilovoltage	Grids
	Collimation
	Object-to-image receptor distance
	Anatomic part
	Contrast media
	Processing

CONTROLLING FACTOR

Kilovoltage is considered the controlling factor for radiographic contrast (Box 4-6). The quality or penetrating power of the x-ray beam has the most direct effect on controlling the desired level of contrast.

Box 4-6 *Controlling Factor for Radiographic Contrast*

The kilovoltage or penetrating power of the x-ray beam controls the desired level of radiographic contrast.

Altering the penetrating power of the x-ray beam affects its absorption and transmission through the anatomic tissue being radiographed. High kilovoltage increases the penetrating power of the x-ray beam and results in lower absorption, more transmission, and fewer density differences in the anatomic tissues; this is described as low contrast (Figure 4-14). When a low kilovoltage is used, the x-ray beam penetration is decreased, resulting in more absorption, less transmission, and more density differences in the tissues; this is described as high contrast (Figure 4-15).

Important Relationship

Kilovoltage and Radiographic Contrast

High kilovoltage creates more densities but with fewer differences, resulting in a low-contrast (long-scale) image. Low kilovoltage creates fewer densities but with greater differences, resulting in a high-contrast (short-scale) image.

The kilovoltage also affects the amount of scatter that occurs during the interaction of the x-ray beam and the anatomic tissue (a result of Compton interactions). A higher kilovoltage increases the percentage of scatter radiation that could interact with the image receptor. Scatter radiation provides no useful information and only adds unwanted density, or fog, on the radiograph. Increasing the amount of fog on a radiograph always decreases the radiographic contrast.

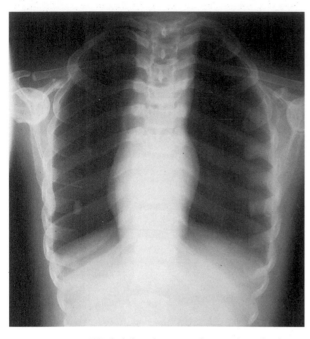

FIGURE 4-14 High-kilovoltage radiograph of chest showing low contrast.

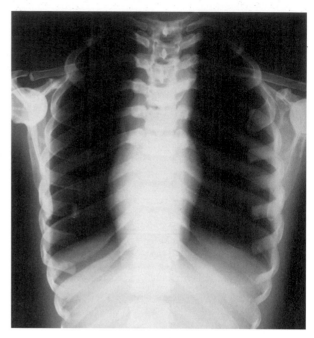

FIGURE 4-15 Low-kilovoltage radiograph of chest showing higher contrast than that in Figure 4-14.

Important Relationship

Kilovoltage, Scatter Radiation, and Radiographic Contrast

Increasing kilovoltage increases the amount of scatter radiation produced and decreases radiographic contrast. Decreasing the kilovoltage decreases scatter production and reduces the amount of fog, therefore increasing radiographic contrast.

The level of radiographic contrast desired, and therefore the kVp level selected, in an image depends on the type and composition of the anatomic tissue, the structures that must be visualized, and to some extent, the diagnostician's preference. These factors make achieving a desired level of radiographic contrast more complex than achieving a desired level of radiographic density.

For most anatomic regions, there is an accepted range of kilovoltage that provides an appropriate level of radiographic contrast. As long as the kilovoltage selected is sufficient to penetrate the anatomic part, the kVp can be further manipulated to alter the radiographic contrast.

Unlike with density errors, radiographs generally are not repeated because of contrast errors. More often, the radiographer evaluates the level of contrast achieved to improve the contrast for additional radiographs or similar circumstances that arise with a different patient.

If a repeat radiograph is necessary and kilovoltage is to be adjusted to either increase or decrease the level of contrast, the 15% rule provides an acceptable method of adjustment. In addition, whenever a 15% change is made in kVp to maintain the same density, the radiographer must adjust the mAs by a factor of 2. Remember that a 15% change in kilovoltage will not produce the same effect across the entire range of kilovoltage used in radiography. A greater increase will be needed for high kilovoltage (90 and above) than for low kilovoltage (below 70).

INFLUENCING FACTORS

Most of the influencing factors affect radiographic contrast by controlling the amount of scatter radiation that reaches the image receptor. Limiting the amount of scatter radiation that reaches the image receptor always increases the radiographic contrast.

Grids

Radiographic grids affect contrast as a result of their absorption of the scatter radiation that exits the patient. A grid is placed between the patient and the image receptor. Much of the scatter radiation exiting the patient will not reach the image receptor when absorbed by a grid (Figure 4-16). The effect of less scatter, or unwanted density (fog), on the image is to increase the radiographic contrast. The

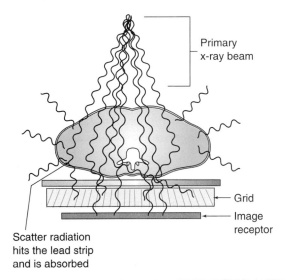

FIGURE 4-16 Much of the scatter radiation toward the image receptor will be absorbed when a grid is used.

more efficient a grid is in absorbing scatter, the greater its effect on radiographic contrast. Grid construction and efficiency are discussed in greater detail in Chapter 6.

Collimation

Changes in the size of the x-ray field affect the amount of the tissue irradiated. A wider field size (decreased collimation) irradiates more tissue and causes more scatter radiation to be produced. The increased amount of scatter radiation reaching the image receptor results in less radiographic contrast. A smaller field size (more collimation) irradiates less tissue and reduces the amount of scatter radiation produced. The decreased amount of scatter radiation reaching the image receptor results in greater radiographic contrast.

The effect of collimation on the radiographic density is more visible when imaging large anatomic areas, performing examinations without a grid, and using a high kilovoltage.

Object-to-Image Receptor Distance

When sufficient distance between the object and image receptor exists, an air gap is created, preventing the scatter radiation from striking the image receptor (Figure 4-17). Whenever the amount of scatter radiation reaching the image receptor is reduced, the radiographic contrast is increased.

The exact amount of object-to-image receptor distance (OID) needed to increase contrast has not been specified. The amount of OID required to increase contrast depends, in part, on the percentage of scatter radiation exiting the patient. For anatomic areas that produce a high percentage of scatter radiation, less OID is needed to increase contrast than for anatomic areas that produce less scatter. In addition, because increased OID also decreases density, the change in contrast may be difficult to perceive.

Important Relationship

Scatter Radiation and Radiographic Contrast

Whenever the amount of scatter radiation reaching the image receptor is reduced, the radiographic contrast is increased (higher contrast).

Anatomic Part

The amount of radiographic contrast achieved is also influenced by the anatomic part to be radiographed. As mentioned earlier, subject contrast is one of the categories of radiographic contrast. The composition and thickness of the tissue and cell compactness affect its absorption characteristics. The absorption characteristics of the anatomic tissue create the range of densities (contrast) produced on a radiograph. Tissues that have a higher atomic number absorb more radiation than those with a lower atomic number.

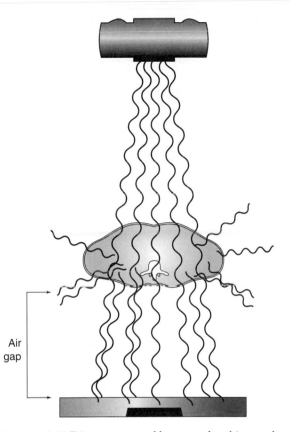

Air
gap

FIGURE 4-17 Distance created between the object and image receptor will reduce the amount of scatter radiation reaching film.

Anatomic structures that have a wide range of tissue composition demonstrate high subject contrast (Figure 4-18). Alternately, anatomic structures that consist of similar type tissue demonstrate low subject contrast (Figure 4-19). The radiographer cannot control the composition of the anatomic part to be radiographed. Changing the kilovoltage alters the absorption characteristics of the tissues irradiated. Knowledge about the absorption characteristics of anatomic tissues and the effect of kilovoltage helps the radiographer to produce a desired level of radiographic contrast.

As the thickness of a given type of anatomic tissue increases, the amount of scatter radiation also increases and radiographic contrast decreases. Using a higher kilovoltage for a thicker part only adds to the increase in scatter radiation. Increased scatter radiation will continue to degrade the quality of the image because it creates fog, which decreases the contrast.

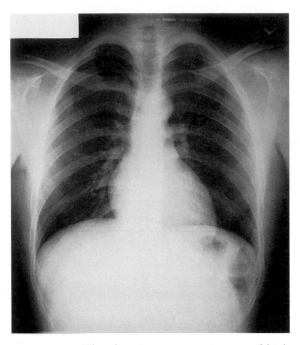

FIGURE 4-18 The chest is an anatomic area of high subject contrast because there is great variation in tissue composition.

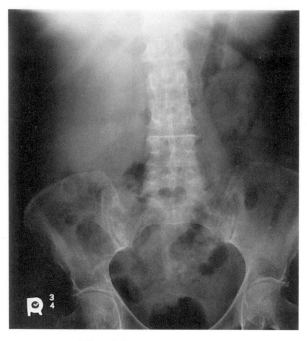

FIGURE 4-19 The abdomen is an anatomic area of low subject contrast because it is made up of similar tissue types.

Important Relationship

Part Thickness and Radiographic Contrast

Increasing part thickness lowers radiographic contrast because of more scatter radiation reaching the image receptor; decreasing part thickness increases radiographic contrast because of less scatter radiation reaching the image receptor.

Tube Filtration

Increasing the amount of tube filtration increases the percentage of higher penetrating x-rays to lower penetrating x-rays. As a result, the x-ray beam has increased energy and can increase the amount of scatter radiation reaching the image receptor. The increased x-ray energy (kV) and scatter production will decrease radiographic contrast. The amount of tube filtration should not vary greatly and therefore small changes will not have a visible effect on radiographic contrast.

Contrast Media

A **contrast medium** (also called *contrast agent*) is used when imaging anatomic tissues that have low subject contrast. A contrast medium is a substance that can be instilled into the body by injection or ingestion. The type of contrast media used will change the absorption characteristics of the tissues by either increasing or decreasing the attenuation of the x-ray beam. Positive contrast agents, such as barium and iodine, have a high atomic number and absorb more x-rays (increase attenuation) than the surrounding tissue (Figure 4-20). Negative contrast agents, such as air, decrease the attenuation of the x-ray beam and transmit more radiation than the surrounding tissue (Figure 4-21). Positive contrast agents produce less radiographic density than the adjacent tissues. Negative contrast agents produce more radiographic density than the adjacent tissues.

Even though negative contrast agents decrease the attenuation characteristics of the part being examined, their use does not require a change in exposure factors. Negative contrast agents can also be used in conjunction with positive contrast agents. Positive contrast media studies require an increase in exposure factors compared to imaging the same part without a positive contrast media.

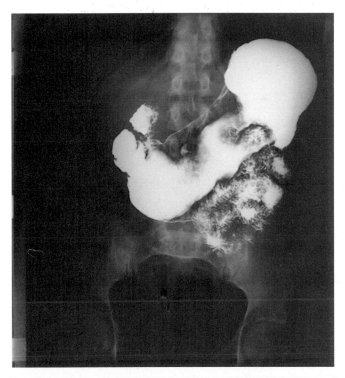

FIGURE 4-20 Radiograph showing decreased density because of the increase in x-ray beam attenuation by use of a positive contrast media agent.

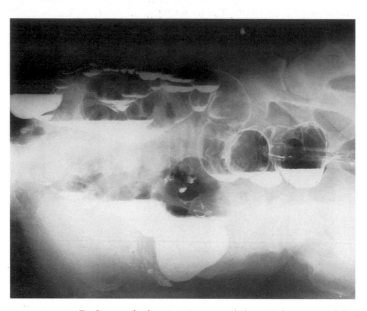

FIGURE 4-21 Radiograph showing increased density because of the decrease in x-ray beam attenuation by use of a negative contrast media agent.

The use of a contrast agent is an effective method of increasing the radiographic contrast when radiographing areas of low subject contrast. Box 4-7 summarizes the photographic factors that control and influence the visibility of recorded detail.

Practical Tip

Selection of Exposure Factors for use with Contrast Media

The radiographer should select a high kVp (90 and above) for barium sulfate studies and a medium kVp (70 to 80) for procedures requiring iodinated solutions.

Box 4-7 *Photographic Factors That Control and Influence the Visibility of Recorded Detail*

Anatomic part	Film-screen system speed
Anode heel effect	Generator output
Collimation	Grids
Contrast media	Kilovoltage
Distance	Milliamperage
Exposure time	Reciprocity law
Film processing	Tube filtration

Digital Imaging

Radiographic contrast is still primarily a result of the kilovoltage and it remains the controlling factor for achieving the desired radiographic contrast on the digital image. In addition, influencing factors such as grids, contrast media, and the composition of the anatomic part affect the subject contrast created on the digital image. Contrast can be further manipulated once the digital image is displayed on a computer monitor. It is important to note that image receptors used in digital imaging are more sensitive to scatter radiation than film-screen receptors. Efforts to minimize the amount of scatter radiation reaching the image receptor discussed in this chapter should be routinely applied during digital imaging. Digital imaging is discussed in more detail in Chapter 12

Important Relationship

Scatter Radiation and Digital Imaging

Digital imaging receptors are more sensitive to scatter radiation than film-screen receptors. Efforts must be routinely made to limit the amount of scatter radiation reaching the digital image receptor.

Exposure Factor Modification

Appropriate exposure factor selection and its modification for variability in the patient are critical to the production of an optimal quality radiograph. The responsibility of creating a quality radiograph lies solely with the radiographer. Thus the radiographer must be able to recognize a multitude of patient and equipment variables and have a thorough understanding of how these variables affect the resulting radiograph in order to make adjustments to produce a quality image.

Pediatric Patients

Pediatric patients are a technical challenge for radiographers for a number of reasons. Pediatric patients, because of their smaller size, require lower values of kilovoltage peak (kVp) and mAs when compared with adults.

Pediatric chest radiography requires the technologist to choose fast exposure times to stop diaphragm motion in patients who cannot or will not voluntarily suspend their breathing. This fast exposure time may eliminate the possibility of using automatic exposure control (AEC) systems for pediatric chest radiography.

Table 4-2 displays the minimum kVp values recommended to penetrate the pediatric chest.

TABLE 4-2	MINIMUM kVp VALUES THAT ARE RECOMMENDED TO PENETRATE THE CHEST IN CHILDREN
Chronological Maturity	**Minimum kVp to Penetrate the Part**
Premature	50
Infant	55
Child	60

Exposure factors used for the adult skull can be used for pediatric patients 6 years of age and older because the bone density of these children has developed to an adult level. However, exposure factors must be modified for patients younger than 6 years of age. It is recommended that the radiographer decrease the kVp value by at least 15% to compensate for this lack of bone density.

For examinations of all other parts of pediatric patients' anatomy, general rules can be used for determining the proper exposure techniques. Recommendations for pediatric exposure techniques, which have been derived from technique charts established for adults, are presented in Table 4-3.

TABLE 4-3	ADAPTING EXPOSURE FACTORS FOR CHILDREN BASED ON EXPOSURE FACTORS FOR ADULTS, EXCLUDING CHEST AND SKULL EXAMINATIONS
Age (in years)	**Exposure Factor Adaptation**
0-5	25% of mAs indicated for adults
6-12	50% of mAs indicated for adults

Projections and Positions

Different radiographic projections and patient positions of the same anatomic part often require modification of exposure factors. For example, an oblique position of the lumbar spine requires more exposure than an anteroposterior (AP) projection because of an increase in the amount of tissue that the primary beam must pass through. However, an oblique ankle requires slightly less exposure than the AP for comparable density.

General guidelines, based on variations in radiographic projection or patient position, can be followed to change exposure factors. When compared to an AP projection, an increase or decrease in the amount of tissue should determine any changes in exposure factors for oblique and lateral patient postions.

Casts and Splints

Casts and splints can be produced with materials that attenuate x-rays differently. Selecting appropriate exposure factors can be challenging because of the wide variation of materials used for these devices. The radiographer should pay close attention to both the type of material and how the cast or splint is used.

Casts

Casts can be produced with either fiberglass or plaster. Fiberglass generally requires no change in exposure factors from the values used for the same anatomic part without a cast.

Plaster presents a problem in terms of exposure factors. Plaster casts require an increase in exposure factors compared with that needed to radiograph the same part without a cast. However, the method and amount of increase in exposure has not been standardized.

One method of approaching the exposure factor conversion is to consider whether the cast is still wet from application or whether it is dry. This approach states that an increase of 2 times the mAs is needed for dry plaster casts and an increase of 3 times the mAs is needed for wet plaster casts. However, Gratale, Turner, and Burns suggest that determining exposure factors for a casted limb on the basis of whether the cast is wet is dry is not relevant. Instead, they demonstrate that it is more important to consider the thickness of the cast.* Thus exposure factor adjustments made for cast materials may be based on the part thickness using a technique chart. For example, if an AP ankle measured through the central ray is 4 inches without the cast and 8 inches with the cast, the radiographer simply increases the mAs to that of an ankle measuring 8 inches to obtain an acceptable radiograph.

Splints

Splints present less of a problem in determining appropriate exposure factors than casts. Inflatable (air) and fiberglass splints do not require any increase in exposure. Wood, aluminum, and solid plastic splints may require that exposure factors be increased, but only if they are in the path of the primary beam. For example, if two pieces of wood are bound to the sides of a lower leg, no increase in exposure is necessary for an AP projection because the splint is not in the path of the primary beam and does not interfere with the radiographic image. Using the same example, if a lateral projection is produced, the splint is in the path of the primary beam and interferes with the radiographic imaging of the part. This necessitates an increase in mAs to produce a properly exposed radiograph.

Body Habitus

Body habitus refers to the general form or build of the body, including size. It is important for the radiographer to consider body habitus when establishing exposure

* From Gratale P, Turner GW, Burns CB: Using the same exposure factors for wet and dry casts, *Radiol Tech* 57(4): 325–329, 1986.

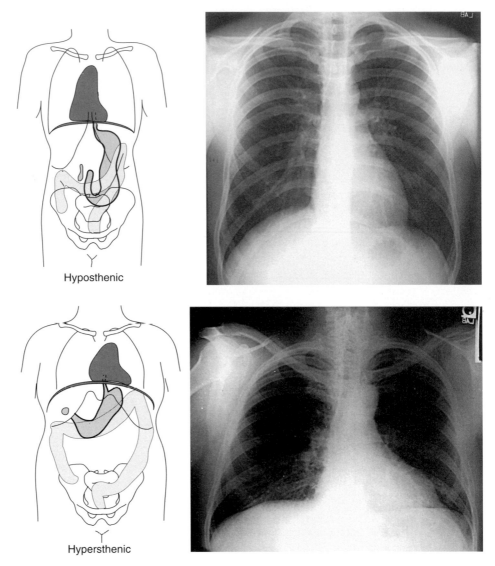

FIGURE 4-22 Four types of body habitus.

From Ballinger P: Merrill's Atlas of Radiographic Positions and Radiologic Procedures, ed. 10, St. Louis, 2003, Mosby.

techniques. There are four types of body habitus: sthenic, hyposthenic, hypersthenic, and asthenic (Figure 4-22).

The sthenic body habitus accounts for approximately 50% of the adult population and is commonly called a *normal* or *average* build. Hyposthenic accounts for approximately 35% of adults and refers to a similar type of body habitus as sthenic, but with a tendency toward a more slender and taller build. Together, the sthenic and

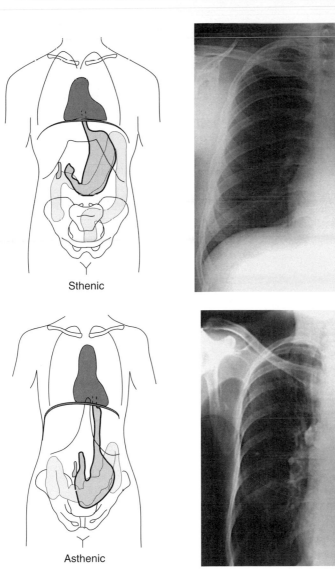

Sthenic

Asthenic

FIGURE 4-22, cont'd
(For legend see previous page)

hyposthenic types of body habitus could, in terms of establishing radiographic techniques, be classified as normal or average of the adult population. This is also convenient because, together, these two types of body habitus account for approximately 85% of adults.

The two remaining types of body habitus are more extreme in terms of size and general occurrence in the adult population. The hypersthenic body habitus, a large, stocky build, accounts for only 5% of adults. These individuals have thicker part sizes compared with sthenic or hyposthenic individuals, so exposure factors for their radiographic examinations are higher.

Asthenic refers to a very slender body habitus and accounts for only 10% of adults. Exposure factors for asthenic individuals are at the low end of technique charts because their respective part sizes are thinner than those of sthenic and hyposthenic individuals.

Pathology

Pathologic conditions that can alter the absorption characteristics of the anatomic part being examined are divided into two categories. Additive diseases are diseases or conditions that increase the absorption characteristics of the part, making the part more difficult to penetrate. Destructive diseases are those diseases or conditions that decrease the absorption characteristics of the part, making the part less difficult to penetrate. Table 4-4 presents a list of additive and destructive diseases. Generally

TABLE 4-4   SOME COMMON ADDITIVE AND DESTRUCTIVE DISEASES AND CONDITIONS BY ANATOMIC AREA

Addictive Conditions	Destructive Conditions
Abdomen	
Aortic aneurysm	Bowel obstruction
Ascites	Free air
Cirrhosis	
Hypertrophy of some organs (e.g., splenomegaly)	
Chest	
Atelectasis	Emphysema
Congestive heart failure	Pneumothorax
Malignancy	
Pleural effusion	
Pneumonia	
Skeleton	
Hydrocephalus	Gout
Metastases (osteoblastic)	Metastases (osteolytic)
Osteochondeoma (exostoses)	Multiple myeloma
Paget's disease (late stage)	Paget's disease (early stage)
	Osteoporosis
Nonspecific Sites	
Abscess	Atrophy
Edema	Emaciation
Sclerosis	Malnutrition

speaking, it is necessary to increase kVp when radiographing parts that have been affected by additive diseases and to decrease kVp when radiographing parts that are affected by destructive diseases.

However, it is not necessary to compensate for all additive and destructive diseases. It is often desirable to image diseases with exposure factors that would normally be used for a specific anatomic part so that the effect of that disease on that part can be visualized clearly. For example, Figure 4-23 demonstrates the first toe radiographed in the AP position. The first metatarsophalangeal joint is affected by osteomyelitis, a destructive disease. It has been radiographed with exposure factors that normally would be used for a toe, without regard for the possible presence of an additive or destructive disease or condition. The normal anatomy of the toe is well visualized, as is the diseased portion.

A similar situation exists with the chest radiograph in Figure 4-24. This patient clearly has pneumonia. The chest was radiographed with exposure factors that normally would be used, without regard for the possibility of pneumonia, an additive disease. The radiograph clearly shows properly exposed normal lung tissue, and yet it demonstrates the pneumonia in an excellent manner. Again, it is not always necessary or desirable to compensate exposure factors for additive or destructive diseases before the initial radiograph.

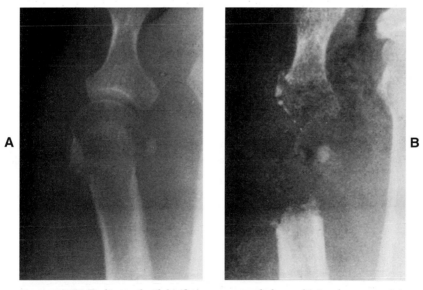

FIGURE 4-23 Radiograph of the first metatarsophalangeal joint demonstrating osteomyelitis. **A,** Soft tissue swelling and periarticular demineralization. **B,** Several weeks later, severe bony destruction.

From Eisenberg R, Dennis C: Comprehensive Radiographic Pathology, ed. 3, St. Louis, 2003, Mosby.

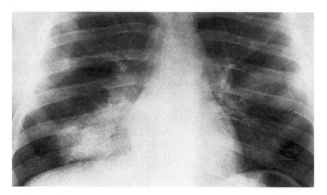

FIGURE 4-24 Radiograph of the chest of a pediatric patient demonstrating pneumonia.

From Eisenberg R, Dennis C: Comprehensive Radiographic Pathology, ed. 3, St. Louis, 2003, Mosby.

When it is necessary or desirable to compensate for additive or destructive diseases or conditions, it is best to make changes in kVp. Changing kVp is fundamentally correct because kVp affects the penetrating ability of the primary beam, and it is the penetrability of the anatomic part that is affected by these particular kinds of diseases or conditions. It is not possible to state an exact amount or percentage of kVp that should be changed because the state or severity of the disease or condition will be different with each patient. However, a minimum change of 15% in kVp is recommended. There are some instances where a change in mAs may be more appropriate to the type of pathology present. For example, if the anatomic area has significant increases in gas, such as in bowel obstruction, a large decrease in mAs would be best.

Soft Tissue

Objects such as small pieces of wood, glass, or swallowed bones are difficult to visualize radiographically using the normal exposure factors for a particular anatomic part. Several situations in which a soft tissue technique may be needed are visualization of the larynx in a young child with the croup, possible foreign body obstruction in the throat, and foreign body location in the extremities (Figure 4-25). Exposure factors must be altered to demonstrate these soft tissues. When the area of interest requires less density to visualize the soft tissue, the mAs should be decreased accordingly.

It is important for the radiographer to determine whether image contrast should be increased or decreased to better visualize the anatomic area of interest. For example, in order to best visualize the airway for the soft tissue neck, radiographic contrast should be increased. However, to visualize a suspected foreign body, it may be necessary to decrease contrast to visualize both bone and soft tissue in the area of

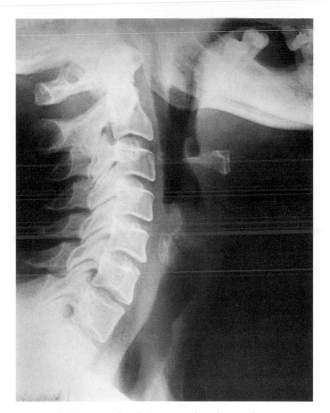

FIGURE 4-25 Lateral soft tissue neck radiograph.
From Ballinger P: Merrill's Atlas of Radiographic Positions and Radiologic Procedures, ed. 10, St. Louis, 2003, Mosby.

interest. The radiographer must determine whether the mAs or the kilovoltage needs adjustment. Soft tissue structures requiring only a decrease in density should be radiographed with decreased mAs, whereas soft tissue structures requiring a higher or lower radiographic contrast should be radiographed with a change in kV. There may also be situations where both the kVp and mAs should be adjusted to alter the contrast yet maintain density.

As mentioned previously, the quality of a radiographic image depends on both the visibility and the sharpness of the recorded detail. Adequate visualization of the anatomic area of interest is just one component of radiographic quality. The ability to visualize an unsharp image is not sufficient for an image of diagnostic quality. The level of sharpness of the recorded image determines the geometric properties of the radiograph (Chapter 5).

The quality of the radiographic image depends on a multitude of variables. Knowledge of these variables and their radiographic effect will assist the radiographer in producing quality radiographs. Table 4-5 provides a chart demonstrating the radiographic effects of the variables discussed in this chapter.

TABLE 4-5 VARIABLES AND THEIR EFFECT ON THE PHOTOGRAPHIC PROPERTIES OF THE RADIOGRAPHIC IMAGE

Radiographic Variables	Density	Contrast
↑ mAs*	↑	0
↓ mAs	↓	0
↑ kVp	↑	↓
↓ kVp	↓	↑
↑ SID	↓	0
↓ SID	↑	0
↑ OID†	↓	↑
↓ OID	↑	↓
↑ Grid ratio	↓	↑
↓ Grid ratio	↑	↓
↑ Film-screen speed	↑	0
↓ Film-screen speed	↓	0
↑ Collimation	↓	↑
↓ Collimation	↑	↓
↑ Focal spot size	0	0
↓ Focal spot size	0	0
↑ Central ray angle	↓	0

mAs, The product of milliamperage and exposure time; *kVp*, kilovoltage peak; *SID*, source-to-image receptor distance; *OID*, object-to-image receptor distance; ↑, increased effect; ↓, decreased effect; *0*, no effect.

*The mAs has no significant effect on contrast as long as densities remain within diagnostic range.

†The amount of OID needed to affect contrast depends on the type of anatomic part being imaged.

FILM CRITIQUE

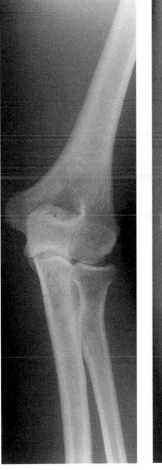

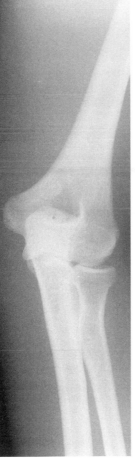

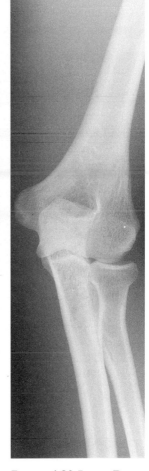

FIGURE 4-26 Image A was produced using 60 kVp, 100 mA at 0.040 s, 100 speed film-screen combination, 40-inch SID, and minimal OID.

FIGURE 4-27 Image B was produced using 60 kVp, 80 mA at 0.025 s, 100 speed film-screen combination, 40-inch SID, and minimal OID.

FIGURE 4-28 Image C was produced using 69 kVp, 160 mA at 0.025 s, 100 speed film-screen combination, 40-inch SID, and minimal OID.

FIGURE 4-29 Image D was produced using 60 kVp, 200 mA at 0.020 s, 100 speed film-screen combination, 40-inch SID, and 3-inch OID.

1. Given that Image A is of optimal quality, discuss the quality of the other images (Figures 4-26, 4-27, 4-28, and 4-29).
2. For each image, evaluate its exposure variables and discuss their effect on the quality of the image (regardless of whether it is apparent on the radiograph).
3. For each image, identify any adjustments that could be made in the exposure factors to produce an image comparable to Image A.

Review Questions

1. A radiograph that needs no improvement is defined as
   A. unacceptable.
   B. optimal.
   C. inadequate.
   D. diagnostic.

2. Factors that affect the visibility of a radiographic image are known as
   A. resolution.
   B. geometric.
   C. densitometric.
   D. photographic.

3. A radiograph that has insufficient density would best be described as
   A. overexposed.
   B. overdeveloped.
   C. underexposed.
   D. underdeveloped.

4. Which of the following is equivalent to doubling the mAs?
   A. Halve the film-screen speed.
   B. Halve the OID.
   C. Double the SID.
   D. Increase kVp by 15%.

5. A radiograph was taken using 65 kVp, 200 mA at 0.10 s. The image needs to be repeated because it is too dark. What exposure technique adjustment would be best?
   A. 65 kVp, 200 mA at 0.05 s
   B. 86 kVp, 200 mA at 0.025 s
   C. 75 kVp, 200 mA at 0.20 s
   D. 55 kVp, 200 mA at 0.10 s

6. What is the relationship between milliamperage and exposure time to maintain density?
   A. Linear
   B. Inverse
   C. Proportional
   D. Direct

7. When repeating a radiograph to correct for a density error, it is recommended to adjust the mAs by a factor of
   A. $\frac{1}{2}$
   B. 2
   C. 3
   D. 4

8. Which of the following factors when *decreased* will *increase* density: (1) grid ratio, (2) focal spot size, or (3) part thickness?
   A. 1 and 2 only
   B. 1 and 3 only
   C. 2 and 3 only
   D. 1, 2, and 3

9. How will radiographic density be affected when the SID is decreased by half?
   A. Increased
   B. Increased by half
   C. Decreased
   D. Decreased by half

10. A radiograph was produced using 85 kVp, 300 mA at 0.2 s. The density is sufficient, but the contrast is too low. Which of the following exposure technique changes would be best to increase the radiographic contrast?
    A. 98 kVp, 300 mA at 0.1 s
    B. 85 kVp, 300 mA at 0.4 s
    C. 72 kVp, 300 mA at 0.4 s
    D. 65 kVp, 300 mA at 0.2 s

11. A radiographic image described as having many shades of gray would be
    A. low density.
    B. low contrast.
    C. high density.
    D. high contrast.

12. The visible differences between adjacent radiographic densities define
    A. fog.
    B. density.
    C. contrast.
    D. resolution.

13. Which of the following will increase radiographic contrast?
    A. Increasing part thickness
    B. Increasing the grid ratio
    C. Increasing the kilovoltage
    D. Increasing filtration

14. Radiographic contrast can be increased by
    A. increasing mAs.
    B. increasing kVp.
    C. decreasing grid ratio.
    D. adding contrast media.

15. What factor has the most direct effect on radiographic contrast?
    A. mAs
    B. SID
    C. Grids
    D. kVp

CHAPTER 5

Radiographic Image Quality: Geometric Properties

1. Define *recorded detail* and discuss the factors affecting geometric unsharpness, receptor unsharpness, and motion unsharpness.

2. Using the geometric unsharpness formula, calculate the changes in the amount of unsharpness when varying SID, OID, and focal spot size.

3. Define *distortion* and discuss the factors that affect both the size and the shape of the recorded image.

4. Calculate the magnification factor and determine the changes in the image and/or object size.

5. Discuss the importance of both the visibility and sharpness of recorded detail in producing a quality radiographic image.

geometric properties
recorded detail
geometric unsharpness
resolution
spatial resolution
contrast resolution
blur

distortion
size distortion/magnification
magnification factor (MF)
source-to-object distance (SOD)
elongation
foreshortening

As discussed in Chapter 4, the quality of a radiographic image depends on both the visibility and the sharpness of the recorded detail. Adequate visualization of the anatomic area of interest is just one component of radiographic quality. The ability to visualize an unsharp image is not sufficient for an image of diagnostic quality. The level of sharpness recorded in the radiograph will be determined by the geometric formation of the image.

Geometric Properties (Sharpness)

The **geometric properties** of a film-screen image refer to the sharpness of structural lines recorded in the radiographic image. A radiographic image cannot be an exact reconstruction of the anatomic structure. Some information is always lost during the process of image formation. It is the radiographer's responsibility to minimize the amount of information lost by accurately manipulating the factors that affect the sharpness of the recorded image. Optimal geometric quality is achieved by maximizing the amount of recorded detail and minimizing the amount of image distortion (Figure 5-1).

Recorded Detail

Recorded detail refers to the distinctness or sharpness of the structural lines that make up the recorded image. The ability of a radiographic image to demonstrate

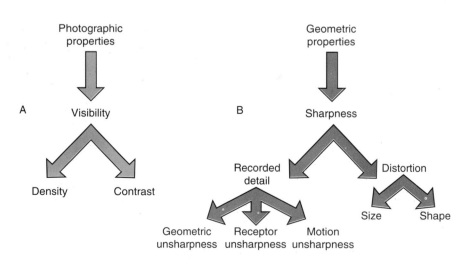

FIGURE 5-1 Geometric properties affecting the sharpness of recorded detail.

sharp lines will determine the quality of the recorded detail. The imaging process makes it impossible to produce a radiographic image without some degree of unsharpness. A radiographic image that has a greater amount of recorded detail will minimize the amount of unsharpness of the anatomic structural lines. The amount of recorded detail is controlled by minimizing geometric unsharpness and receptor unsharpness and by eliminating motion unsharpness.

GEOMETRIC UNSHARPNESS

The amount of **geometric unsharpness** is a result of the relationship among the size of the focal spot, SID, and OID (Figure 5-2). Manipulating each variable individually or in combination alters the amount of unsharpness recorded in the image.

Focal Spot Size

The physical dimensions of the focal spot on the anode target in x-ray tubes used in standard radiographic applications usually range from 0.5 to 1.2 mm. Focal spot size is determined by the filament size. When the radiographer selects a particular focal spot size, he or she is actually selecting a filament size that will be energized during x-ray production. On the control panel the radiographer can select whether to use a small focal spot size or a large one. Small focal spot sizes are usually 0.5 or 0.6 mm in size, and large focal spot sizes are usually 1.0 or 1.2 mm in size. Focal spot size is an

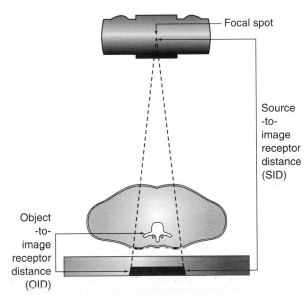

FIGURE 5-2 Geometric unsharpness is influenced by the relationship among focal spot, SID, and OID.

important consideration for the radiographer to make because focal spot size controls recorded detail (Figure 5-3).

Important Relationship

Focal Spot Size and Recorded Detail

As focal spot size increases, unsharpness increases and recorded detail decreases; as focal spot size decreases, unsharpness decreases and recorded detail increases.

In general, the smallest focal spot size available should be used for every exposure. Unfortunately, exposure is limited with a small focal spot size. When a small focal spot is used, the heat created during the x-ray exposure is concentrated in a smaller area and could cause tube damage. The radiographer must weigh the importance of improved recorded detail for a particular examination or anatomic part against the amount of exposure used. Modern radiographic x-ray generators are equipped with safety circuits that prevent an exposure from being made if that exposure will exceed the tube loading capacity for the focal spot size selected. Repeated exposures made just under the limit over a long period can still jeopardize the life of the x-ray tube.

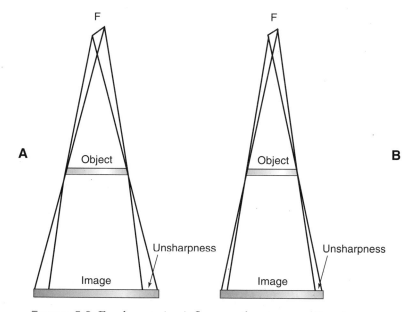

FIGURE 5-3 Focal spot size influences the amount of unsharpness recorded in the image. As focal spot size changes, so does the amount of unsharpness. **A,** Larger focal spot. **B,** Smaller focal spot.

Practical Tip

Selecting Focal Spot Size

The radiographer should select the smallest focal spot size, considering the amount of x-ray exposure used and the amount of recorded detail required for the radiographic examination.

Distance

As discussed previously, distance plays an important role in radiographic imaging. Just as the intensity of the x-ray beam is altered when changing the distance between the source and object or the object and receptor, so is the amount of unsharpness recorded on the image. Because of the diverging properties of the x-ray beam, a geometric relationship exists among the source of x-rays, the object, and the image receptor (Figure 5-4).

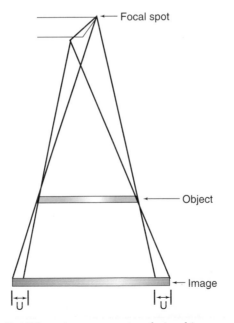

FIGURE 5-4 There is a geometric relationship among the x-ray source, object, and image receptor. *U,* Unsharpness.

Figure 5-5 demonstrates that when the SID is increased, the amount of image unsharpness is decreased. As the distance between the source and image receptor increases, the diverging x-rays become more perpendicular to the object radiographed.

Important Relationship

SID, Unsharpness, and Recorded Detail

Increasing the SID decreases the amount of unsharpness and increases the amount of recorded detail in the image, whereas decreasing the SID increases the amount of unsharpness and decreases the recorded detail.

Standard distances for SID are used in radiography to accommodate equipment limitations. Except for chest and cervical spine radiography, a 40-inch (100-cm) or 48-inch (122-cm) SID is the standard.

In addition to SID, the OID also affects the amount of unsharpness recorded on the image. Optimal recorded detail is achieved when the OID is zero. Unfortunately, this cannot realistically be achieved in radiographic imaging because there is always some distance created between the area of interest and the image receptor.

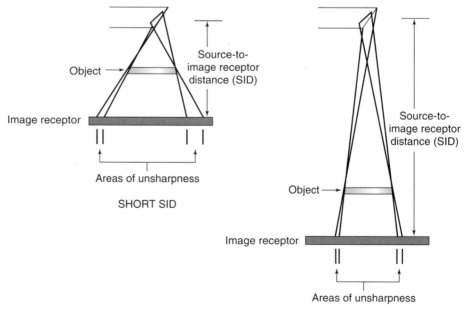

FIGURE 5-5 Increasing source-to-image receptor distance decreases the amount of geometric unsharpness.

As the exit beam leaves the patient, it continues to diverge. When distance is created between the area of interest and the image receptor, the diverging exit beam records increased unsharpness within the image (Figure 5-6).

Important Relationship

OID, Unsharpness, and Recorded Detail

Increasing the OID increases the amount of unsharpness and decreases the recorded detail, whereas decreasing the amount of OID decreases the amount of unsharpness and increases the recorded detail.

The distance between the area of interest and the image receptor has the greatest effect on the amount of geometric unsharpness recorded. When possible, the distance between the area of interest and the image receptor should be kept to a minimum. When a film-screen image receptor is used and placed in a radiographic table, some amount of increased OID will always occur. It is the radiographer's responsibility to position the area of interest as close to the image receptor as possible to minimize the amount of unsharpness recorded.

The relationship among the variables of focal spot size and distance can be demonstrated mathematically by the geometric unsharpness formula (Box 5-1).

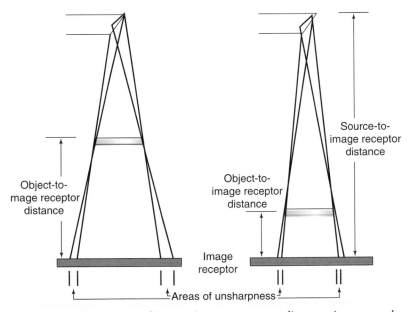

FIGURE 5-6 Increasing object-to-image receptor distance increases the amount of geometric unsharpness.

Box 5-1 *Geometric Unsharpness Formula*

$$\text{Geometric unsharpness} = \frac{\text{Focal spot size} \times \text{OID}}{\text{SOD}}$$

where
Focal spot size = Dimensions of the effective focal spot in millimeters (mm)
OID   = The distance between the object (area of interest) and the image receptor
SOD   = The distance between the focal spot (source) and object (area of interest)
SOD   = SID − OID

When calculating the amount of geometric unsharpness, the radiographer must keep the distance measurement in the same units (i.e., inches or centimeters). This will cancel the units and result in the geometric unsharpness unit of millimeters.

The unit of geometric unsharpness provides a method of mathematically comparing the amount of unsharpness present for a given focal spot size and distance.

 X *Mathematical Application*

Calculating Geometric Unsharpness

The amount of geometric unsharpness can be calculated for each of the following images to determine which image has more geometric unsharpness.

Image 1	**Image 2**
Focal spot size = 0.6 mm	Focal spot size = 1.2 mm
SID = 40 inches	SID = 56 inches
OID = 0.25 inch	OID = 4.0 inches

Image 1

$$\frac{0.6 \text{ mm} \times 0.25 \text{ inch}}{39.75 \text{ inches}}; \frac{0.15}{39.75}$$

Image 2

$$\frac{1.2 \text{ mm} \times 4 \text{ inches}}{52 \text{ inches}}; \frac{4.8}{52}$$

Geometric unsharpness of Image 1 = 0.004 mm
Geometric unsharpness of Image 2 = 0.09 mm

Image 2 has the greater amount of unsharpness.

Although minimizing geometric unsharpness is important, the radiographer also must consider the effect of these variables on the x-ray tube. The smallest focal spot size may not be the best choice when radiographing the lateral lumbar spine, nor is the amount of recorded detail as important in this anatomic region when compared with extremities. In addition, using a 72-inch SID is not practical for most radiographic studies, although it is justified when imaging the chest or lateral cervical spine.

Practical Tip

Minimizing Geometric Unsharpness

The radiographer should select the smallest focal spot size when maximal recorded detail is important; he or she should also consider the amount of heat load within the x-ray tube. In addition, the radiographer should select the standard SID when OID is minimal. When increased OID is unavoidable, SID should be increased slightly to compensate.

The radiographer has the most control over the amount of unsharpness recorded in the image by manipulating the focal spot size, selecting the appropriate SID, and maintaining minimal OID.

IMAGE RECEPTOR UNSHARPNESS

The type of device used to record the image also affects the amount of unsharpness recorded in the image. In conventional radiography, various intensifying screen-film combinations have created a complex system of image receptors. Variations in the construction and composition of the intensifying screen combined with different types of radiographic film affect not only the photographic properties of the image but also its geometric properties.

One of the significant advancements in image receptors has been their ability to limit the amount of x-rays needed to produce a visible image. The ability to reduce the exposure to the patient has been at a cost to the quality of the image, most often in recorded detail.

As mentioned in the section on film-screen systems' effect on density, the higher the relative speed of the film-screen system, the fewer x-rays needed to create the image. The changes that are needed to increase the relative speed of the film-screen system will also decrease the amount of recorded detail within the radiographic image. The composition and construction of intensifying film-screen systems are discussed in more detail in Chapter 7.

Important Relationship

Intensifying Film-Screen Speed, Recorded Detail, and Unsharpness

Increasing the relative speed of the intensifying film-screen system decreases the recorded detail and increases the amount of unsharpness recorded in the image. Decreasing the relative speed of the intensifying film-screen system increases the recorded detail and decreases the amount of unsharpness recorded in the image.

Because the radiographic film normally is placed between two intensifying screens, any distance that is created between the film and screen causes increased unsharpness to be recorded in the image. Poor film-screen contact creates an area of unsharpness because the light emitted from the intensifying screen phosphor crystal diverges from its origin. When there is distance between the film and phosphor crystal, the light spread causes unsharp structural lines to be recorded in the image (Figure 5-7). It is important to maintain good film-screen contact to maximize recorded detail. If good film-screen contact cannot be maintained, the screen must be repaired or discarded.

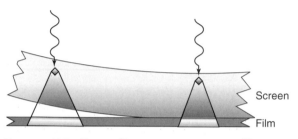

FIGURE 5-7 Poor film-screen contact will cause increased unsharpness.

RESOLUTION

Recorded detail can be measured and is expressed as resolution. **Resolution** is the ability of the imaging system to resolve or distinguish between two adjacent structures. Resolution can be expressed in the unit of line pairs per millimeter (Lp/mm). A resolution test pattern is a device used to record and measure line pairs (Figure 5-8). The greater the number of line pairs per millimeter resolved, the greater the resolution and recorded detail.

In the space of 1 mm, the number of line pairs resolved determines the amount of recorded detail. Each line pair is made up of a line and a space. Visual acuity of the human eye is limited to the ability to discern approximately 5-Lp/mm. At this level, each line measures 0.1 mm and a line pair measures 0.2 mm. An imaging system that can resolve a greater number of line pairs within 1 mm (e.g., 8 to 10 Lp/mm) is said to have improved recorded detail. The average human eye would not be able to distinguish this improved recorded detail. However, when resolution is measured below 5 Lp/mm (e.g., 2 to 3 Lp/mm), the reduced recorded detail can be discerned.

Resolution can be considered a combined result of both spatial and contrast resolution. These terms have become more important since the introduction of digital imaging. **Spatial resolution** refers to the smallest detail that can be detected in an image. Film-screen imaging systems have excellent spatial resolution. **Contrast**

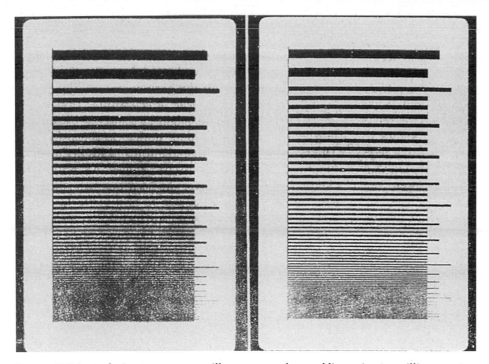

FIGURE 5-8 A resolution test pattern will measure and record line pairs per millimeter.
From Mosby's instructional radiographic series: radiographic imaging, St Louis, 1998, Mosby.

resolution refers to the ability of the imaging system to distinguish between small objects having similar subject contrast. Digital imaging systems have improved contrast resolution when compared to film-screen systems.

Sharpness of recorded detail and visibility of recorded detail have typically been discussed as two separate qualities of the radiographic image. Generally this remains true, except when imaging small anatomic structures. A small anatomic structure is best visualized when its density varies significantly from the background. If unsharpness is increased, the visibility of small anatomic detail is compromised. An increase in the amount of unsharpness recorded on the image decreases the contrast of small anatomic structures, thereby reducing the overall visibility of recorded detail. The spreading of the structural lines with increased unsharpness decreases the density differences between the structural lines of the area of interest and the background. As a result, the difference in density between the area of interest and the background becomes less (low contrast) and the visibility of the anatomic structure is reduced (Figure 5-9).

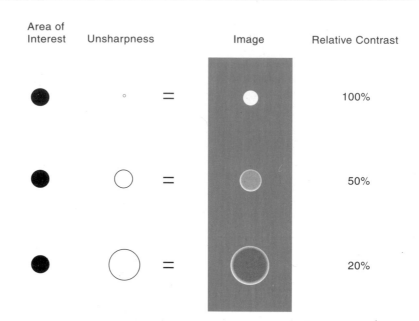

| Area of Interest | Unsharpness | | Image | Relative Contrast |

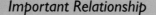

FIGURE 5-9 Unsharpness and image contrast. Increasing the amount of unsharpness will decrease the density difference (contrast) between the area of interest and its surrounding background. *Modified from Sprawls P:* Physical Principles of Medical Imaging, *2nd ed, New York, 1993, Aspen Publishers.*

MOTION UNSHARPNESS

Motion unsharpness has the most detrimental effect on the recorded detail of the radiographic image. Motion of the tube, part, or image receptor causes a profound decrease in recorded detail. Motion must not just be decreased; it must be eliminated.

Important Relationship

Motion and Recorded Detail

Motion of the tube, patient, part, or image receptor greatly decreases recorded detail.

Unsharpness resulting from patient motion, known as **blur,** is the most detrimental factor to maximizing recorded detail (Figure 5-10). Unsharpness resulting from patient motion can be classified as voluntary (within the patient's control) or involuntary (outside of patient's control, such as peristalsis). Most motion on radiographs results from the patient moving during the exposure. The radiographer can control patient motion to some degree. Patients who are least likely to cooperate, and therefore move, are pediatric patients, those with conditions such as Parkinson's disease that cause involuntary shaking, and those who are otherwise unwilling or unable to cooperate, such as intoxicated or traumatized patients.

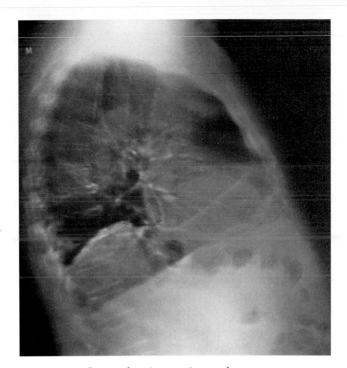

FIGURE 5-10 Image showing motion unsharpness.
From Mosby's instructional radiographic series: radiographic imaging, St Louis, 1998, Mosby.

If a patient needs to be physically held, it is generally recommended that the holder not be a person who routinely is exposed to x-rays. The holder should always wear lead shielding and, if female, be evaluated for the possibility of pregnancy before making the exposure.

A less typical type of motion unsharpness can be caused by equipment, such as undesirable motion of the tube, table, or image receptor. Motion of the tube or image receptor is not very likely because tube assemblies and film trays have locks that are easily used by the radiographer.

Practical Tip

Eliminating Motion

Patient motion can be controlled by the following:

1. Using short exposure times compensated for by higher mA
2. Providing clear instructions for the patient to assist in immobilization
3. Using physical immobilization, such as sandbags, tape, or other devices, as deemed necessary

Distortion

Distortion results from the radiographic misrepresentation of either the size (magnification) or shape of the anatomic part. When the image is distorted, recorded detail is also reduced.

SIZE DISTORTION (MAGNIFICATION)

The term **size distortion/magnification** refers to an increase in the object's image size compared with its true, or actual, size. Radiographic images of objects are always magnified in terms of the true object size. The distances used (SID and OID) play an important role in minimizing the amount of size distortion of the radiographic image.

Object-to-Image Receptor Distance

Magnification of the true object will occur because there is always some OID during radiography. OID is directly related to magnification.

Important Relationship

OID and Size Distortion

As OID increases, size distortion (magnification) increases; as OID decreases, size distortion (magnification) decreases.

Because radiographers produce radiographs of three-dimensional objects, some size distortion always occurs as a result of OID. Even if the object is in close contact with the image receptor, some part of the object will be farther away from the image receptor than other parts of the object. Those parts of the object that are farther away from the image receptor will be represented radiographically with more size distortion than parts of the object that are closer to the image receptor.

Figure 5-11 shows how two objects of the same size are demonstrated radiographically using a short OID and a long OID. Notice how a long OID produces more size distortion than a short OID.

Practical Tip

Minimizing OID

The radiographer should always try to minimize OID as much as possible to reduce size distortion (magnification). Within the protocol of the examination, it is always best to try to position the area of interest closest to the image receptor to minimize size distortion of that area.

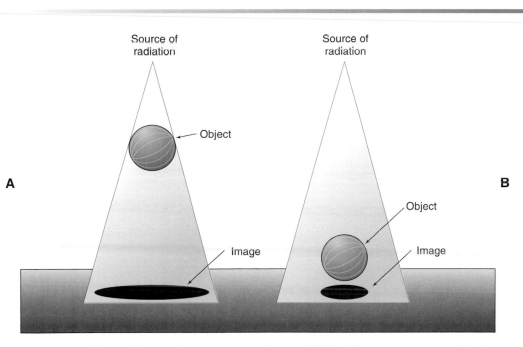

FIGURE 5-11 A long object-to-image receptor distance (OID) will create more magnification than a short OID. The image in **A** is larger than that in **B** because the object is farther from the image receptor.

Source-to-Image Receptor Distance

SID also influences the total amount of size distortion represented on a radiograph. Although OID has the greatest effect on size distortion, SID is still an important factor for the radiographer to control in order to minimize size distortion. SID is inversely related to magnification.

Important Relationship

SID and Size Distortion

As SID increases, size distortion (magnification) decreases; as SID decreases, size distortion (magnification) increases.

Figure 5-12 illustrates how a long SID produces less size distortion than a short SID. In some situations it is difficult to minimize OID because of factors or conditions outside of the radiographer's control. In these instances size distortion can still be reduced by increasing SID.

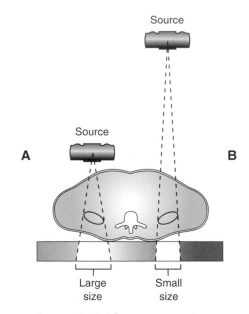

FIGURE 5-12 A long source-to-image receptor distance (SID) will create less magnification than a short SID. The image in **A** is larger than that in **B** because the object is closer to the source.

Calculating Magnification

To observe the effect of distance on size distortion, it is necessary to consider the magnification factor. The **magnification factor (MF)** indicates how much size distortion or magnification is demonstrated on a radiograph. The MF can be expressed mathematically by the following formula:

$$MF = \frac{SID}{SOD}$$

SOD represents **source-to-object distance,** which refers to the distance from the x-ray source (focal spot) to the object being radiographed. SOD can be expressed mathematically as follows:

$$SOD = SID - OID$$

SOD is also demonstrated in Figure 5-13.

An MF of 1.00 indicates no magnification. No magnification means that the size of the radiographic image matches the true object size. This is an impossible situation because some magnification exists on every radiograph. An MF greater than 1.0 can be expressed as a percentage of magnification.

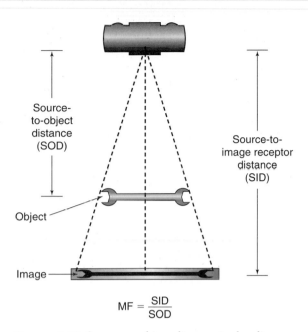

$$MF = \frac{SID}{SOD}$$

FIGURE 5-13 Source-to-object distance is the distance between the source of x-ray and the object radiographed.

✗ Mathematical Application

The Magnification Factor

A posteroanterior (PA) projection of the chest was produced with an SID of 72 inches and an OID of 3 inches. What is the MF?

$$MF = \frac{72 \text{ inches}}{69 \text{ inches}}$$

$$MF = 1.044$$

In the case of the Mathematical Application for MF, an MF of 1.044 means that the image is 4.4% larger than the true object size. It should be noted that the MF computed here is a minimum. A 3-inch OID implies that the anterior surface of the patient's chest was 3 inches away from the image receptor for a PA projection. Anatomy that is posterior to the anterior chest wall is farther away from the image receptor and will be magnified even more.

Once the MF is known, the object size can then be determined. This requires the use of another formula:

$$\text{Object size} = \frac{\text{Image size}}{MF}$$

It may be helpful to know the measurement of the true object size in comparison to its size on a radiographic image.

X *Mathematical Application*

Determining Object Size

On a PA chest film taken with an SID of 72 inches and an OID of 3 inches (SOD is equal to 69 inches), the size of a round lesion in the right lung measures 1.5 inches in diameter on the radiograph. The MF has been determined to be 1.044. What is the object size of this lesion?

$$\text{Object size} = \frac{1.5 \text{ inches}}{1.044}$$

$$\text{Object size} = 1.44 \text{ inches}$$

Perhaps the most practical use of these formulas is to observe how changing the SID and OID affects the image size. Size distortion or magnification can be increased by decreasing the SID or by increasing the OID. This increase in magnification can be demonstrated mathematically by using the MF, then calculating the change in the size of the object on the radiographic image.

SHAPE DISTORTION

In addition to size distortion, objects that are being imaged can also be misrepresented radiographically by distortion of their shape. Shape distortion can appear in two different ways radiographically: elongation or foreshortening. **Elongation** refers to images of objects that appear longer than the true objects. **Foreshortening** refers to images that appear shorter than the true objects. Examples of elongation and foreshortening can be seen in Figure 5-14.

Shape distortion can occur from inaccurate central ray (CR) alignment of the tube, the part being radiographed, or the image receptor. Any misalignment of the CR among these three factors—tube, part, or image receptor—will alter the shape of the part recorded on the film.

For example, Figure 5-15, *A* and *B*, demonstrates shape distortion when the anatomic part and image receptor are misaligned. In addition, shape distortion becomes more obvious if the CR of the primary beam is not directed to enter or exit the anatomy as required for the particular projection or position (off centering). This happens because the path of individual photons in the primary beam become more divergent as the distance increases from the CR. The radiographer must properly control alignment of the tube, part, and image receptor, and he or she must properly direct the CR to minimize shape distortion.

Sometimes, shape distortion is used to an advantage in particular projections or positions. CR angulation, for example, is sometimes required to elongate a part so

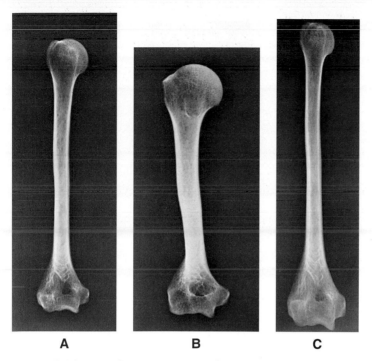

FIGURE 5-14 A, No distortion. **B,** Foreshortened. **C,** Elongated.

From Mosby's instructional radiographic series: radiographic imaging, St Louis, 1998, Mosby.

that a particular anatomic structure can be visualized better. Also, CR angulation is sometimes required to eliminate superimposition of objects that normally would obstruct visualization of the area of interest. In general, shape distortion is not a necessary or desirable characteristic of radiographs.

Practical Tip

Minimizing Shape Distortion

Elongation and foreshortening can be minimized by ensuring the proper CR alignment of the following:

1. X-ray tube
2. Part
3. Image receptor
4. Entry or exit point of the CR

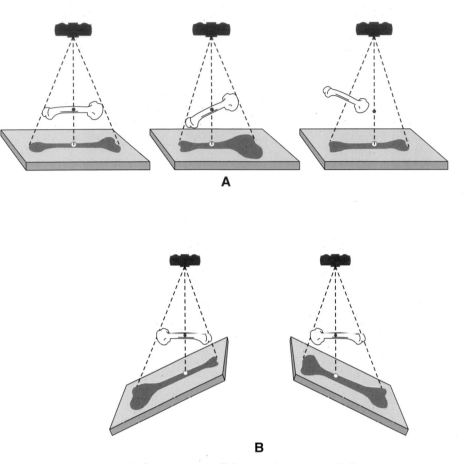

FIGURE 5-15 A, Part not parallel to image receptor. **B,** Image receptor not parallel to part.

From Mosby's instructional radiographic series: radiographic imaging, St Louis, 1998, Mosby.

The quality of the radiographic image depends on many variables. Knowledge of these variables and their radiographic effect assists the radiographer in producing quality radiographs. Table 5-1 provides a chart demonstrating the radiographic effects of the variables discussed in this chapter and Chapter 4.

Digital Imaging

The geometric factors that affect image quality are also applicable to digital imaging systems. Focal spot size, SID, and OID alter the amount of geometric unsharpness recorded in the digital image. Any motion, which results from patient movement or the equipment, also decreases the recorded detail of the image.

TABLE 5-1   **VARIABLES AND THEIR EFFECT ON BOTH THE PHOTOGRAPHIC AND GEOMETRIC PROPERTIES OF THE RADIOGRAPHIC IMAGE**

Radiographic Variables	Photographic Properties Recorded		Geometric Properties	
	Density	Contrast	Detail	Distortion
↑ mAs*	↑	0	0	0
↓ mAs	↓	0	0	0
↑ kVp	↑	↓	0	0
↓ kVp	↓	↑	0	0
↑ SID	↓	0	↑	↓
↓ SID	↑	0	↓	↑
↑ OID†	↓	↑	↓	↑
↓ OID	↑	↓	↑	↓
↑ Grid ratio	↓	↑	0	0
↓ Grid ratio	↑	↓	0	0
↑ Film-screen speed	↑	0	↓	0
↓ Film-screen speed	↓	0	↑	0
↑ Collimation	↓	↑	0	0
↓ Collimation	↑	↓	0	0
↑ Focal spot size	0	0	↓	0
↓ Focal spot size	0	0	↑	0
↑ Central ray angle	↓	0	↓	↑

mAs, The product of milliamperage and exposure time; kVp, kilovoltage peak; SID, source-to-image receptor distance; OID, object-to-image receptor distance; ↑, increased effect; ↓, decreased effect; 0, no effect.
*The mAs has no significant effect on contrast as long as densities remain within diagnostic range.
†The amount of OID needed to affect contrast depends on the type of anatomic part being imaged.

    All of the factors that determine the amount of image distortion are equally important for digital and film-screen imaging. Both SID and OID determine the amount of magnification of the anatomic structures on the image. In addition, improper alignment of the central ray, anatomic part, image receptor, or a combination of these components distorts the shape of the digital image.

FILM CRITIQUE

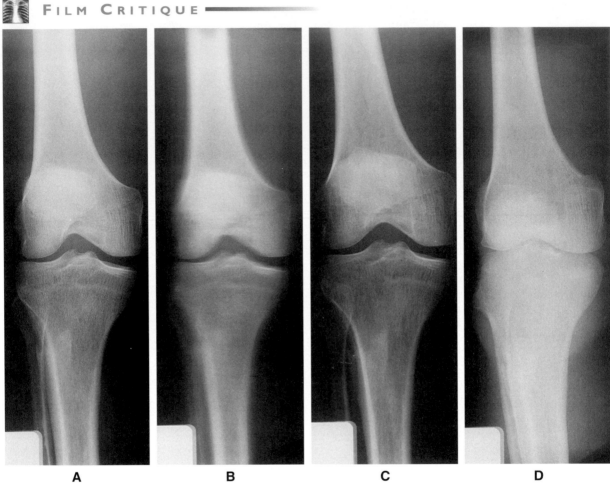

A

FIGURE 5-16 Image **A** was produced using 65 kVp, 100 mA at 0.10 s, 400 speed film-screen combination, 40-inch SID, central ray perpendicular, small focal spot size, and minimal OID.

B

FIGURE 5-17 Image **B** was produced using 65 kVp, 10 mA at 1.0 s. 400 speed film-screen combination, 40-inch SID, central ray perpendicular, small focal spot size, and minimal OID.

C

FIGURE 5-18 Image **C** was produced using 65 kVp, 500 mA at 0.20 s, 400 speed film-screen combination, 35-inch SID, central ray perpendicular, large focal spot size, and 2-inch OID.

D

FIGURE 5-19 Image **D** was produced using 65 kVp, 100 mA at 0.064 s, 600 speed film-screen combination, 44-inch SID, central ray angled 40 degrees caudad, small focal spot size, and minimal OID.

1. Given Image A is of optimal quality, discuss the quality of the other images (Figures 5-16, 5-17, 5-18 and 5-19).
2. For each image, evaluate its exposure variables and discuss their effect on the quality of the image (regardless of whether it is apparent on the radiograph).
3. For each image, identify any adjustments that could be made in the exposure factors to produce an image comparable to Image A.

Review Questions

1. Recorded detail is defined as
   A. accuracy of structural lines recorded.
   B. visibility of the structural lines.
   C. misrepresentation of the shape of the structural lines.
   D. amount of structural lines.

2. The relationship between focal spot size and distance results in
   A. receptor unsharpness.
   B. motion blur.
   C. geometric unsharpness.
   D. shape distortion.

3. Increasing the SID will
   A. increase unsharpness.
   B. increase distortion.
   C. increase magnification.
   D. increase recorded detail.

4. Decreasing the OID will
   A. increase unsharpness.
   B. increase distortion.
   C. increase magnification.
   D. increase recorded detail.

5. The ability of the imaging system to distinguish between two adjacent structures defines
   A. blur.
   B. resolution.
   C. distortion.
   D. acuity.

6. The amount of unsharpness created using a focal spot of 0.6 mm, an SID of 36 inches, and an OID of 3 inches is
   A. 0.005
   B. 0.055
   C. 0.567
   D. 0.635

7. What is the image size of a part measuring 2.5 cm using an SID of 100 cm, an OID of 5 cm, and a focal spot of 1.25 mm?
   A. 2.37 cm
   B. 2.50 cm
   C. 2.63 cm
   D. 2.75 cm

8. Using a larger focal spot size has what effect on the radiographic image?
   A. Decreases density
   B. Decreases contrast
   C. Decreases distortion
   D. Decreases recorded detail

9. Shape distortion can be created by
   A. angling the CR.
   B. decreasing the SID.
   C. increasing the focal spot size.
   D. increasing the OID.

10. Which of the following has the most detrimental effect on the recorded detail of the image?
    A. Large focal spot size
    B. Increased OID
    C. Motion
    D. Magnification

CHAPTER 6

Scatter Control

Controlling the amount of scatter radiation that reaches the image receptor (IR) is essential in creating an optimal quality image. Scatter radiation is detrimental to radiographic quality because it adds unwanted density to the image without adding any patient information. Therefore the radiographer must act to minimize the amount of scatter radiation reaching the image receptor.

Beam-restricting devices and radiographic grids are tools the radiographer can use to limit the amount of scatter radiation reaching the IR. Beam-restricting devices decrease the x-ray beam field size and the amount of tissue irradiated, thereby reducing the amount of scatter radiation produced. Radiographic grids are used to improve the radiographic image quality by absorbing scatter radiation that exits the patient.

Scatter Radiation

Scatter radiation, as described in Chapter 3, is primarily the result of the Compton interaction, in which the incoming x-ray photon loses energy and changes direction. There are two major factors that affect the amount of scatter radiation reaching the image receptor: kVp and the volume of tissue irradiated. The volume of tissue depends on the thickness of the part as well as the x-ray beam field size. Using higher kVp's or increasing the volume of tissue irradiated results in increased scatter radiation reaching the IR.

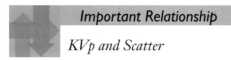

Important Relationship

KVp and Scatter

The amount of scatter produced within the patient depends, in part, on the kVp selected. Exams using higher kVp's produce a greater proportion of scattered x-rays as compared to low kVp exams.

Important Relationship

X-ray Beam Field Size, Thickness of the Part, and Scatter

The larger the x-ray beam field size, the greater the amount of scatter radiation produced. The thicker the part being imaged, the greater the amount of scatter radiation produced.

Important Relationship

Volume of Tissue Irradiated and Scatter

The volume of tissue irradiated is affected by both the part thickness and the x-ray beam field size. Therefore the greater the volume of tissue irradiated, because of either or both factors, the greater the amount of scatter radiation produced.

Practical Tip

The Role of the Radiographer

In performing radiographic exams, the radiographer both selects the kVp and adjusts the beam restriction. It is up to each radiographer to use the kVp appropriate to the exam and to limit the x-ray beam field size to the anatomic area of interest.

Beam restriction serves two purposes: limiting patient exposure and reducing the amount of scatter radiation produced within the patient.

Beam Restriction

The unrestricted primary beam is cone shaped and projects a round field on the patient and image receptor (Figure 6-1). If not restricted in some way, the primary beam will go beyond the boundaries of the image receptor, resulting in unnecessary patient exposure. Any time the x-ray field extends beyond the anatomic area of interest, the patient is receiving unnecessary exposure. Limiting the x-ray beam field size is accomplished with a beam-restricting device. Located just below the x-ray tube housing, the **beam restricting device** changes the shape and size of the primary beam.

The terms **beam restriction** and **collimation** are used interchangeably; they refer to a decrease in the size of the projected radiation field. The term *collimation* is used more often than the term *beam restriction* because collimators are the most popular type of beam-restricting device. Increasing collimation means decreasing field size, and decreasing collimation means increasing field size.

Important Relationship

Beam Restriction and Patient Dose

As beam restriction or collimation increases, field size decreases and patient dose decreases. As beam restriction or collimation decreases, field size increases and patient dose increases.

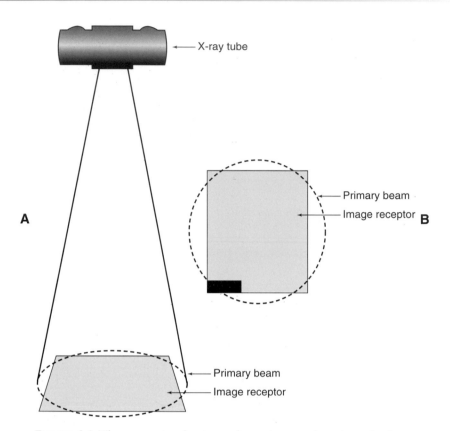

FIGURE 6-1 The unrestricted primary beam is cone shaped, projecting a circular field. **A,** Side view. **B,** View from above.

Beam Restriction and Scatter Radiation

In addition to decreasing patient dose, beam-restricting devices also reduce the amount of scatter radiation that is produced within the patient, reducing the amount of scatter the image receptor is exposed to, and thereby increasing the radiographic contrast.

The relationship between collimation (field size) and quantity of scatter radiation is illustrated in Figure 6-2. As stated previously, collimation means decreasing the size of the projected field, so increasing collimation means decreasing field size, and decreasing collimation means increasing field size.

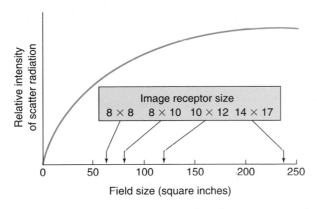

FIGURE 6-2 As field size increases, the relative quantity of scatter radiation increases.

Important Relationship

Collimation and Scatter Radiation

As collimation increases, the field size decreases and the quantity of scatter radiation decreases; as collimation decreases, the field size increases and the quantity of scatter radiation increases.

COLLIMATION AND CONTRAST

Because collimation decreases the x-ray beam field size, less scatter radiation is produced within the patient. Therefore less scatter radiation reaches the image receptor. As described in Chapter 4, this affects the radiographic contrast.

Important Relationship

Collimation and Radiographic Contrast

As collimation increases, the quantity of scatter radiation decreases, and radiographic contrast increases; as collimation decreases, the quantity of scatter radiation increases, and radiographic contrast decreases.

COMPENSATING FOR COLLIMATION

An increase in collimation also affects the number of x-ray photons reaching the IR and radiographic density (film-screen). Increasing collimation decreases the number of photons that strike the patient and image receptor and decreases the amount of scatter radiation produced. Therefore exposure factors may need to be changed when increasing collimation.

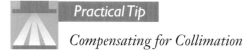

Important Relationship

Collimation and Radiographic Density

As collimation increases, radiographic density decreases; as collimation decreases, radiographic density increases.

Practical Tip

Compensating for Collimation

When collimating significantly (changing from an 11- × 14-inch field size to a small, 4-inch-diameter cone), the radiographer must increase exposure to compensate for the loss of density that otherwise occurs. The kilovoltage peak (kVp) value should not be increased because it results in decreased contrast. To change density only, mAs should be changed.

It has been recommended that significant collimation requires an increase in as much as 30% to 50% of the mAs (as described and calculated in Chapter 2) to compensate for the loss in density that occurs because of collimation.

Important relationships regarding the restriction of the primary beam are summarized in Table 6-1.

TABLE 6-1   RESTRICTING THE PRIMARY BEAM

Increased Factor	Result
Collimation	Patient dose **decreases.**
	Scatter radiation **decreases.**
	Radiographic contrast **increases.**
	Radiographic density **decreases.**
Field size	Patient dose **increases.**
	Scatter radiation **increases.**
	Radiographic contrast **decreases.**
	Radiographic density **increases.**

Types of Beam-Restricting Devices

Several types of beam-restricting devices are available, which differ in sophistication and utility. All beam-restricting devices are made of metal or a combination of metals that readily absorb x-rays.

APERTURE DIAPHRAGMS

The simplest type of beam-restricting device is the aperture diaphragm. An **aperture diaphragm** is a flat piece of lead (diaphragm) that has a hole (aperture) in it. Commercially made aperture diaphragms are available (Figure 6-3), as are those that are homemade (hospital-made) for purposes specific to a radiographic unit. Aperture diaphragms are easy to use. They slide into slots at the bottom of a collimator, or they can be taped directly onto the tube housing in the absence of a collimator. An aperture diaphragm can be made by cutting rubberized lead into the size needed to create the diaphragm and cutting the center to create the shape and size of the aperture.

Although the aperture's size and shape can be changed, the aperture cannot be adjusted from the designed size. Therefore the projected field size is not adjustable. In addition, because of the aperture's proximity to the radiation source (focal spot), a large area of unsharpness surrounds the radiographic image (Figure 6-4). Although

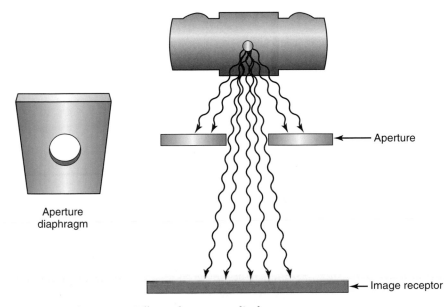

Aperture
diaphragm

Aperture

Image receptor

FIGURE 6-3 A commercially made aperture diaphragm.

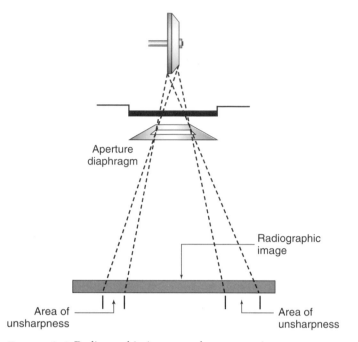

FIGURE 6-4 Radiographic image unsharpness using an aperture diaphragm.

aperture diaphragms are still used in some applications, their use is not as widespread as that of other types of beam-restricting devices.

CONES AND CYLINDERS

Cones and cylinders are shaped differently (Figure 6-5), but they have many of the same attributes. A **cone** or **cylinder** is essentially an aperture diaphragm that has an extended flange attached to it. The flange can vary in length and can be shaped as either a cone or a cylinder. The flange can also be made to telescope, thereby increasing its total length (Figure 6-6). Like aperture diaphragms, cones and cylinders are easy to use. They simply attach to the slots in the bottom of a collimator. Cones and cylinders limit unsharpness surrounding the radiographic image more than aperture diaphragms do, with cylinders accomplishing this task slightly better than cones (Figure 6-7). However, they are limited in terms of the sizes that are available, and they are not necessarily interchangeable among tube housings. Cones have a particular disadvantage compared with cylinders. If the angle of the flange of the cone is greater than the angle of divergence of the primary beam, the base plate or aperture diaphragm of the cone is the only metal actually restricting the primary beam. Therefore cylinders generally are more useful than cones. Cones and cylinders are almost always made to produce a circular projected field, and they can be used to advantage for particular radiographic procedures (Figure 6-8).

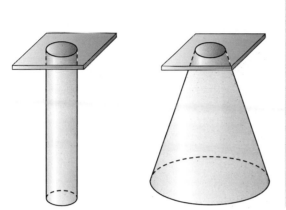

FIGURE 6-5 A, A cylinder. **B**, A cone.

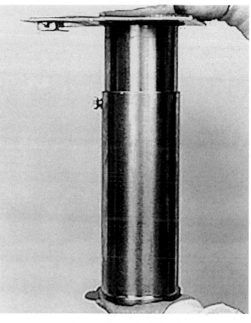

FIGURE 6-6 A telescoping cylinder.

From Mosby's radiographic instructional series: radiographic imaging, St Louis, 1998, Mosby.

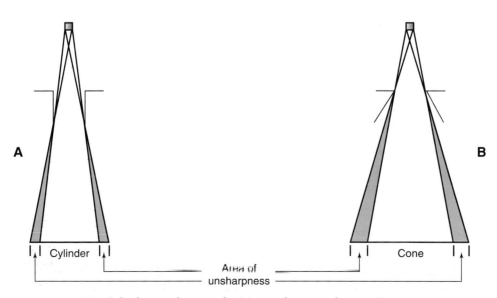

FIGURE 6-7 A, Cylinders are better at limiting unsharpness than are, **B**, cones.

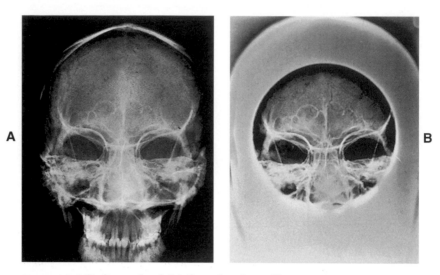

FIGURE 6-8 Radiograph of the frontal and maxillary sinuses, **A,** not using a cone and, **B,** using a cone.

From Mosby's radiographic instructional series: radiographic imaging, St Louis, 1998, Mosby.

COLLIMATORS

The most sophisticated, useful, and accepted type of beam-restricting device is the collimator. Collimators are considered the best type of beam-restricting device available for radiography. Beam restriction accomplished with the use of a collimator is referred to as *collimation.* The terms *collimation* and *beam restriction* are used interchangeably.

A **collimator** has two sets of adjustable lead shutters (Figure 6-9). Each set of shutters consists of longitudinal and lateral leaves or blades, each with its own control. This makes the collimator adjustable in terms of its ability to produce projected fields of varying sizes. The field shape produced by a collimator is always rectangular or square unless an aperture diaphragm, cone, or cylinder is used in conjunction with it. Collimators are equipped with a white light source and a mirror to project a light field onto the patient. This light is intended to accurately indicate where the primary x-ray beam will be projected during exposure. In case of failure of this light, an x-ray field measurement guide (Figure 6-10) is present on the front of the collimator. It indicates the projected field size based on the adjusted size of the collimator opening at particular source-to-image receptor distances (SIDs). This helps ensure that the radiographer does not open the collimator to produce a field that is larger than the image receptor. Another problem that may occur is the lack of accuracy of the light field. The mirror that reflects the light down toward the patient or the light bulb itself could be slightly out of position, projecting a light field that inaccurately indicates where the primary beam will be projected. There is a means of testing the accuracy of this light field and the location of the center of projected beam.

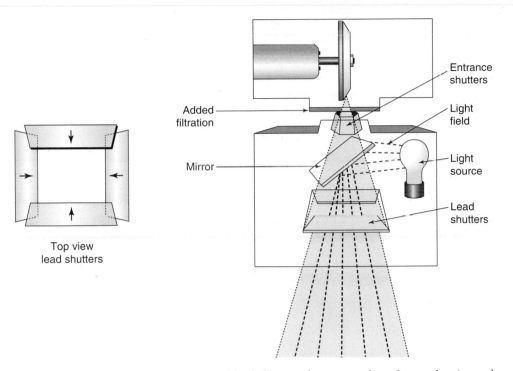

Top view
lead shutters

FIGURE 6-9 Collimators have two sets of lead shutters that are used to change the size and shape of the primary beam.

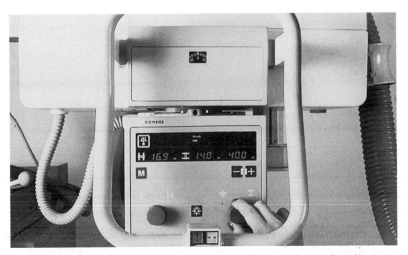

FIGURE 6-10 The x-ray field measurement guide on the front of a collimator.

A plastic template with crosshairs is affixed to the bottom of the collimator to indicate where the center of the primary beam—the central ray—will be directed. This is of great assistance to the radiographer in accurately centering the x-ray field to the patient.

AUTOMATIC COLLIMATORS

Automatic collimators are also called *positive beam-limiting devices,* or *PBLs.* An **automatic collimator,** or **positive beam-limiting device,** automatically limits the size and shape of the primary beam to the size and shape of the image receptor. For a number of years, automatic collimators were required by U.S. federal law on all new radiographic installations. This law has since been rescinded, and automatic collimators are no longer a requirement on any radiographic equipment. However, they are still widely used. Automatic collimators mechanically adjust the primary beam size and shape to that of the image receptor when the IR is placed in the Bucky tray, just below the table top. Automatic collimation makes it difficult for the radiographer to increase the size of the primary beam to a field larger than the image receptor, which would result in increasing the patient's radiation exposure. PBL devices were seen as a way of protecting patients from overexposure to radiation. However, it should be noted that automatic collimators have an override mechanism that allows the radiographer to disengage this feature.

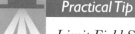

Practical Tip

Limit Field Size to Image Receptor Size

The size of the projected radiation field should never exceed the size of the image receptor. This will ensure patient protection from excessive radiation exposure while also improving image quality.

Radiographic Grids

The radiographic grid was invented in 1913 by Gustave Bucky. Approximately $\frac{1}{4}$-inch thick and ranging from 8×10 inches to 17×17 inches, a **grid** is a device that has very thin interspaced lead strips intended to absorb scatter radiation emitted from the patient before it strikes the image receptor. Placed between the patient and the image receptor, grids are invaluable in the practice of radiography. They work well to improve radiographic contrast but are not without drawbacks. As will be discussed later in this chapter, using a grid requires additional mAs, resulting in a higher patient dose. Therefore grids are typically used only when the anatomic part is 10 cm or greater in thickness, and more than 60 kVp is needed for the exam.

When to use a grid

A grid should be used when the anatomic part being imaged is 10 cm or more (typically the size of an adult knee) and more than 60 kVp is appropriate for the exam.

As scatter radiation leaves the patient, a significant amount of it is directed at the image receptor. As stated previously, scatter radiation exposure is detrimental to radiographic quality because it adds unwanted density to the radiograph without adding any patient information. Scatter radiation decreases radiographic contrast. Ideally, grids would absorb, or clean up, all scattered photons directed toward the image receptor and would allow all transmitted photons emitted from the patient to pass from the patient to the image receptor. Unfortunately, this does not happen (Figure 6-11). When used properly, however, grids can greatly increase the contrast of the radiographic image.

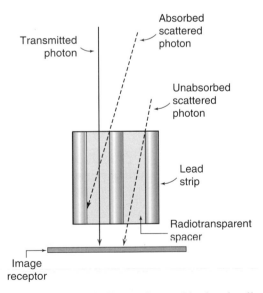

FIGURE 6-11 Ideally, grids would absorb all scattered radiation and allow all transmitted photons to reach the film. In reality, however, some scattered photons pass through to the film, and some transmitted photons are absorbed.

> *Important Relationship*
>
> *Scatter Radiation and Image Quality*
>
> Scatter radiation adds unwanted density to the radiograph and decreases image quality.

Grid Construction

Grids contain thin lead strips or lines that have a precise height, thickness, and space between them. Radiolucent **interspace material** separates the lead lines. Interspace material typically is made of aluminum. The lead lines and interspace material of the grid are covered by an aluminum front and back panel.

Grid construction can be described by grid frequency and grid ratio. **Grid frequency** expresses the number of lead lines per unit length, in inches, centimeters, or both. Grid frequencies can range in value from 25 to 45 lines/cm (60 to 110 lines/inch). A typical value for grid frequency might be 40 lines/cm or 103 lines/inch. Another way of describing grid construction is by its grid ratio. **Grid ratio** is defined as the ratio of the height of the lead strips to the distance between them (Figure 6-12). Grid ratio can also be expressed mathematically as follows:

$$\text{Grid ratio} = h/D$$

where *h* is the height of the lead strips and *D* is the distance between them.

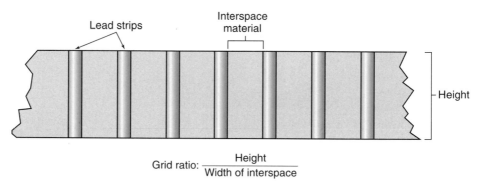

FIGURE **6-12** Grid ratio is the ratio of the height of the lead strips to the distance between them.

Calculating Grid Ratio

What is the grid ratio when the lead strips are 3.2 mm high and separated by 0.2 mm?

$$\text{Grid ratio} = h/D$$

$$\text{Grid ratio} = \frac{3.2}{0.2}$$

$$= 16 \text{ or } 16{:}1$$

Grid ratios range from 4:1 to 16:1. High-ratio grids remove, or clean up, more scatter radiation than lower-ratio grids and thus further increase radiographic contrast.

Important Relationship

Grid Ratio and Radiographic Contrast

As grid ratio increases, scatter cleanup improves and radiographic contrast increases; as grid ratio decreases, scatter cleanup is less effective and radiographic contrast decreases.

Information about a grid's construction is contained on a label placed on the tube side of the grid. This label usually states the type of interspace material used, grid frequency, grid ratio, grid size, and information about the range of SIDs that can be used with the grid. The radiographer should read this information before using the grid because these factors influence grid performance and image quality.

GRID PATTERN

Grid pattern refers to the linear pattern of the lead lines of a grid. Two types of grid pattern exist: linear and crossed or cross-hatched. A **linear grid** has lead lines that run in only one direction (Figure 6-13). Linear grids are the most popular in terms of grid pattern because they allow angulation of the x-ray tube along the length of the lead lines. A **crossed** or **cross-hatched grid** has lead lines that run at a right angle to one another (Figure 6-14). Crossed grids remove more scattered photons than linear

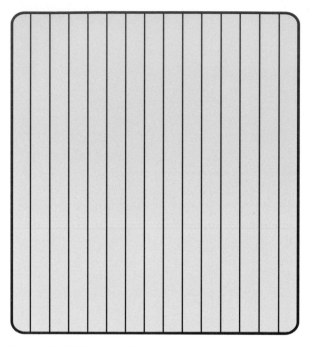

FIGURE 6-13 Linear grid pattern.

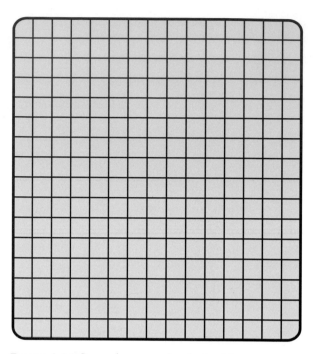

FIGURE 6-14 Crossed or cross-hatched grid pattern.

grids because they contain more lead strips, oriented in two directions. However, applications are limited with a crossed grid because the x-ray tube cannot be angled in any direction without producing grid cutoff (i.e., absorption of the transmitted x-rays). Grid cutoff is undesirable and is discussed later in this chapter.

GRID FOCUS

Grid focus refers to the orientation of the lead lines to one another. Two types of grid focus exist: parallel (non-focused) and focused. A **parallel** or **non-focused grid** has lead lines that run parallel to one another (Figure 6-15). Parallel grids are used primarily in fluoroscopy and mobile imaging. A **focused grid** has lead lines that are angled to approximately match the angle of divergence of the primary beam (Figure 6-16). The advantage of focused grids compared with parallel grids is that focused grids allow more transmitted photons to reach the image receptor. As seen in Figure 6-17, transmitted photons are more likely to pass through a focused grid to reach the IR than they are to pass through a parallel grid.

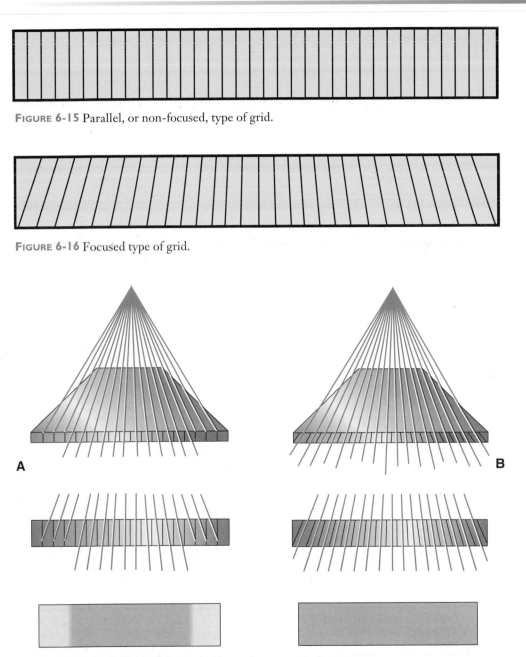

FIGURE 6-15 Parallel, or non-focused, type of grid.

FIGURE 6-16 Focused type of grid.

A

B

FIGURE 6-17 Comparison of transmitted photons passing through, **A,** a parallel grid and, **B,** a focused grid.

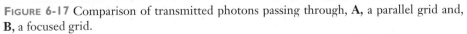

![Important Relationship icon]

Important Relationship

Focused versus Parallel Grids

Focused grids have lead lines that are angled to approximately match the divergence of the primary beam. Thus focused grids allow more transmitted photons to reach the image receptor than parallel grids.

As seen in Figure 6-18, if imaginary lines were drawn from each of the lead lines in a linear focused grid, these lines would meet to form an imaginary point, called the **convergent point**. If points were connected along the length of the grid they would form an imaginary line, called the **convergent line.** Both the convergent line and convergent point are important because they determine the focal distance of a focused grid. The **focal distance** (sometimes referred to as grid radius) is the distance between the grid and the convergent line or point. The focal distance is important because it is used to determine the focal range of a focused grid. The **focal range** is the recommended range of SIDs that can be used with a focused grid. The convergent line or point always falls within the focal range (Figure 6-19). For example, a common focal range is 36 to 42 inches, with a focal distance of 40 inches. Another common focal range is 66 to 74 inches, with a focal distance of 72 inches.

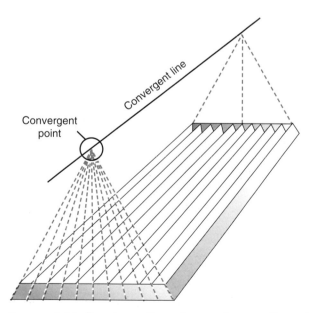

FIGURE 6-18 Imaginary lines drawn above a linear focused grid from each lead strip meet to form a convergent point; the points form a convergent line.

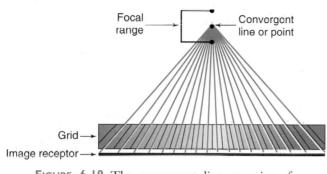

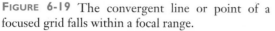

FIGURE 6-19 The convergent line or point of a focused grid falls within a focal range.

Because the lead lines in a parallel grid are not angled, they have a focal range extending from a minimum SID to infinity.

Types of Grids

Grids are available for use by the radiographer in several forms and can be stationary or moving. Stationary, non-moving grids include the wafer grid, grid cassette, and grid cap. A **wafer grid** matches the size of the cassette and is used by placing it on top of the image receptor. Wafer grids typically are taped to the image receptor to prevent them from sliding during the radiographic procedure. A **grid cassette** is an image receptor that has a grid permanently mounted to its front surface. A **grid cap** contains a permanently mounted grid and allows the image receptor to slide in behind it. This is useful because the grid is secure, and many image receptors can be interchanged behind the grid before processing the image.

STATIONARY AND RECIPROCATING GRIDS

When grids are stationary it is possible to closely examine and see the grid lines on the radiographic image. Slightly moving the grid during the x-ray exposure blurs the grid lines

Moving or reciprocating grids are part of the **Bucky**, more accurately called the Potter-Bucky diaphragm. Located directly below the radiographic tabletop, the grid is found just above the tray that holds the image receptor. Grid motion is controlled electrically by the x-ray exposure switch. The grid moves back and forth in a lateral direction over the image receptor during the entire exposure. These grids typically have dimensions of 17 × 17 inches so that a 14 × 17 inch cassette can be positioned under the grid either lengthwise or crosswise, depending on the examination requirements.

Grid Performance

The purpose of using grids in radiography is to increase radiographic contrast. Thus the best measure of how well a grid performs is the contrast improvement factor. The **contrast improvement factor** is expressed mathematically as follows:

$$K = \frac{\text{Radiographic contrast with a grid}}{\text{Radiographic contrast without a grid}}$$

where *K* signifies the contrast improvement factor. This is a fundamental formula in terms of quality assurance applications.

In addition to improving contrast by cleaning up scatter, grids reduce the total amount of x-rays reaching the image receptor and therefore reduce the density (film-screen). The better the grid is at absorbing scattered photons, such as with a higher ratio grid, the fewer the photons reaching the image receptor. To compensate for this reduction, additional mAs must be used to produce optimal images. The **grid conversion factor (GCF),** or **Bucky factor**, can be used to determine the adjustment in mAs needed when changing from using a grid to non-grid (or vice versa) or for changing to grids with different grid ratios.

The GCF can be expressed mathematically as:

$$GCF = \frac{\text{mAs with the grid}}{\text{mAs without the grid}}$$

Important Relationship

Grid Ratio and Radiographic Density

As grid ratio increases, radiographic density decreases; as grid ratio decreases, radiographic density increases.

Table 6-2 presents specific grid ratios and grid conversion factors. When a grid is added to the image receptor, mAs must be increased by the factors indicated to maintain radiographic density, or the same number of x-ray photons reaching the IR. This requires multiplication by the GCF for the particular grid ratio.

TABLE 6-2   **THE BUCKY FACTOR/GRID CONVERSION FACTOR (GCF)**

Grid Ratio	Bucky Factor/GCF
5:1	2
6:1	3
8:1	4
12:1	5
16:1	6

✗ Mathematical Application

Adding a Grid

If a radiographer produced a knee radiograph with a non-grid exposure using 10 mAs and next wanted to use an 8:1 grid, what mAs should be used to produce a radiograph with the same density?

Nongrid exposure = 10 mAs

GCF (for 8:1 grid) = 4 (from Table 6-2)

$$GCF = \frac{\text{mAs with the grid}}{\text{mAs without the grid}}$$

$$4 = \frac{\text{mAs with the grid}}{10}$$

$$40 = \text{mAs with the grid}$$

When adding an 8:1 grid, the mAs must be increased by a factor of 4, in this case to 40 mAs.

Likewise, if a radiographer chooses to not use a grid during a procedure, but only knows the appropriate mAs when a grid is used, the mAs must be decreased by the GCF. This requires division by the GCF for the particular grid ratio.

✗ Mathematical Application

Removing a Grid

If a radiographer produced a knee radiograph using a 16:1 grid and 60 mAs, and on the next exposure wanted to use a non-grid exposure, what mAs should be used to produce a radiograph with the same density?

Grid exposure = 60 mAs

GCF (for 16:1 grid) = 6 (from Table 6-2)

$$GCF = \frac{\text{mAs with the grid}}{\text{mAs without the grid}}$$

$$6 = \frac{60}{\text{mAs without the grid}}$$

$$10 = \text{mAs without the grid}$$

When removing a 16:1 grid, the mAs must be decreased by a factor of 6, in this case to 10 mAs.

The GCF is also useful when changing between grids with different grid ratios. When changing from one grid ratio to another, the following formula should be used to adjust the mAs:

$$\frac{mAs_1}{mAs_2} = \frac{GCF_1}{GCF_2}$$

✗ Mathematical Application

Increasing the Grid Ratio

If a radiographer performed a routine portable abdomen exam using 30 mAs with a 6:1 grid, what mAs should be used if a 12:1 grid is used?

Exposure 1: 30 mAs, 6:1 grid, GCF = 3

Exposure 2: _____ mAs, 12:1 grid, GCF = 5

$$\frac{mAs_1}{mAs_2} = \frac{GCF_1}{GCF_2}$$

$$\frac{30}{mAs_2} = \frac{3}{5}$$

$$mAs_2 = 50$$

Increasing the grid ratio requires additional mAs.

✗ Mathematical Application

Decreasing the Grid Ratio

If a radiographer used 40 mAs with an 8:1 grid, what mAs should be used with a 5:1 grid in order to produce the same density?

Exposure 1: 40 mAs, 8:1 grid, GCF = 4

Exposure 2: _____ mAs, 5:1 grid, GCF = 2

$$\frac{mAs_1}{mAs_2} = \frac{GCF_1}{GCF_2}$$

$$\frac{40}{mAs_2} = \frac{4}{2}$$

$$mAs_2 = 20$$

Decreasing the grid ratio requires less mAs.

The increase in mAs required to maintain density on the radiograph results in an increase in patient dose. This increase in patient dose is significant, as the numbers for the GCF indicate.

It is important to remember that patient dose is increased because of the following:

1. Using a grid compared with not using a grid
2. Using a higher ratio grid

> ### Important Relationship
>
> *Grid Ratio and Patient Dose*

As grid ratio increases, patient dose increases; as grid ratio decreases, patient dose decreases.

Grid Cutoff

In addition to the disadvantage of increased patient dose associated with grid use, another disadvantage is the possibility of grid cutoff. **Grid cutoff** is defined as a decrease in the number of transmitted photons that reach the image receptor because of some misalignment of the grid. The primary radiographic effect of grid cutoff is a further reduction in the number of photons reaching the IR, and a decrease in radiographic density. Grid cutoff often requires that the radiographer repeat the radiograph, thereby increasing patient dose yet again. Grid ratio has a significant impact on grid cutoff, with higher grid ratios resulting in more potential cutoff.

Types of Grid Cutoff Errors

Grid cutoff can occur as a result of four types of errors in grid use. To reduce or eliminate grid cutoff, the radiographer must have a thorough understanding of the importance of proper grid alignment in relation to the image receptor and x-ray tube.

UPSIDE DOWN FOCUSED

Upside down focused grid cutoff occurs when a focused grid is placed upside down on the image receptor, resulting in the grid lines going opposite the angle of divergence of the x-ray beam. This appears radiographically as significant loss of density along the edges of the image (Figure 6-20). Photons easily pass through the center of the grid because the lead lines are perpendicular to the image receptor surface. Lead lines that are more peripheral to the center are angled more and thus absorb the transmitted photons.

FIGURE 6-20 Radiograph produced with an upside down focused grid.

Important Relationship

Upside Down Focused Grids and Grid Cutoff

Placing a focused grid upside down on the image receptor causes the lateral edges of the radiograph to be very light (underexposed).

Practical Tip

Using upside down focused grid

Upside down focused grid error is easily avoided because every focused grid should have a label indicating "Tube Side." This side of the grid should always face the tube, away from the image receptor.

OFF-LEVEL

Off-level grid cutoff results when the x-ray beam is angled across the lead strips. It is the most common type of cutoff and can occur from either the tube or grid being angled (Figure 6-21). Off-level grid cutoff can often be seen with mobile radiographic studies or horizontal beam exams and appears as a loss of density across the entire image. This type of grid cutoff is the only type that occurs with both focused and parallel grids

Important Relationship

Off –Level Error and Grid Cutoff

Angling the x-ray tube across the grid lines or angling the grid itself during exposure produces an overall decrease in density on the radiograph.

OFF-CENTER

Also called lateral decentering, off-center grid cutoff occurs when the central ray of the x-ray beam is not aligned from side to side with the center of a focused grid.

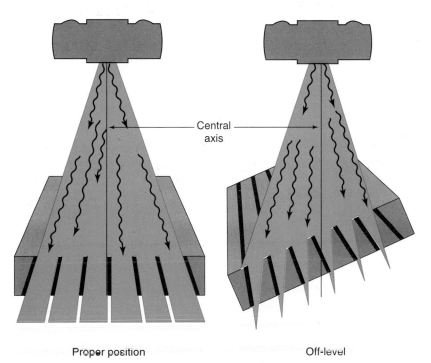

Proper position   Off-level

FIGURE 6-21 An off-level grid can cause grid cutoff.

Because of the arrangement of the lead lines of the focused grid, the divergence of the primary beam does not match the angle of these lead strips when not centered (Figure 6-22). Off-center grid cutoff appears radiographically as an overall loss of density (Figure 6-23).

> ### Important Relationship
>
> *Off-Center Error and Grid Cutoff*

If the center of the x-ray beam is not aligned from side to side with the center of a focused grid, grid cutoff will occur.

OFF-FOCUS

Off-focus grid cutoff occurs when using an SID outside of the recommended focal range. Grid cutoff occurs if the SID is less than or greater than the focal range. Both appear the same radiographically as a loss of density at the periphery of the film (Figure 6-24).

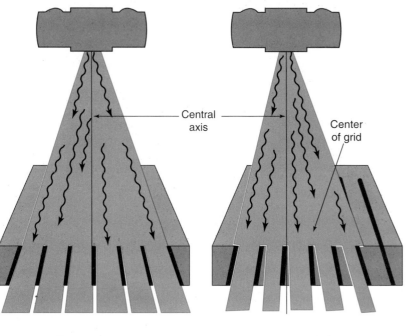

Proper position   Off-center

FIGURE 6-22 Centering to one side of a focused grid can cause off-center grid cutoff.

FIGURE 6-23 Radiograph demonstrating off-center grid cutoff.

FIGURE 6-24 Radiograph demonstrating off-focus grid cutoff.

Important Relationship

Off-Focus Error and Grid Cutoff

Using an SID outside of the focal range creates a loss of density at the periphery of the radiograph.

Table 6-3 summarizes important relationships regarding the use of radiographic grids.

TABLE 6-3   **RADIOGRAPHIC GRIDS**

Increased Factor	Result
Grid ratio*	Contrast **increases.** Patient dose **increases.** The likelihood of grid cutoff **increases.**

*mAs adjusted to maintain density.

Grid Usage

There are a number of factors for the radiographer to consider when deciding on the type of grid, if any, to be used for an exam. Although quite efficient at preventing scatter radiation from reaching the image receptor, grids are not appropriate for all exams. When appropriate, selection of a grid involves consideration of contrast improvement, patient dose, and the likelihood of grid cutoff. Radiographers typically choose between parallel and focused grids, high and low-ratio grids, grids with different focal ranges, and whether or not to use a grid at all.

As indicated earlier, the choice of whether or not to use a grid is based on the kVp necessary for the exam and the thickness of the part. Parts 10 cm or larger, together with kVp higher than 60, produce enough scatter to necessitate the use of a grid. The next question is which grid to use. There is no single best grid for all situations. A 16:1 focused grid will provide excellent contrast improvement, but the patient's dose will be high and the radiographer must ensure that the grid and x-ray tube are perfectly aligned to prevent grid cutoff. The 5:1 parallel grid will do a mediocre job of scatter cleanup, especially at kVp's above 80. However, the patient dose will be significantly lower, and the radiographer need not be concerned with cutoff caused by being off-center, SID used, or having the grid upside-down. Selection between grids with different focal ranges depends on the radiographic exam. Supine abdomen studies should use a grid that includes 40 inches in the focal range; upright chest studies should have grids that include 72 inches. In general, most radiographic rooms use a 10:1 or 12:1 focused grid, which provides a compromise between contrast improvement and patient dose. Stationary grids, for mobile exams in particular, may be lower ratio, parallel, or both to allow the radiographer greater positioning latitude.

Practical Tip

Grid Selection

Grids differ from one another in performance, especially in the areas of grid ratio and focal distance. Before using a grid, the radiographer must determine the grid ratio so that the appropriate exposure factors can be selected. Also, the radiographer must be aware of the focal range of focused grids so that the appropriate SID is selected. Box 6-1 lists attributes of the grid typically used in radiography.

Box 6-1 *The Typical Grid*

Is linear instead of crossed
Is focused instead of parallel
Is of mid-ratio (8:1 to 12:1)
Has a focal range that includes an SID of 40 or 72 inches

The Air Gap Technique

Whereas the radiographer may use the grid most often to prevent scatter from reaching the image receptor, the grid is not the only available tool. Although limited in its usefulness, the air gap technique provides another method for limiting the scatter reaching the IR. The **air gap technique** is based on the simple concept that much of the scatter will miss the image receptor if there is increased distance between the patient and image receptor (increased OID) (Figure 6-25). The greater the gap, the greater the reduction in scatter reaching the IR. Similar to a grid, contrast is increased, the number of photons reaching the IR is reduced because less scatter reaches the IR, and the mAs must be increased to compensate.

The air gap technique is limited in its usefulness because the necessary OID results in decreased recorded detail. To overcome this increase in unsharpness, an increase in SID is required, which may not always be feasible. The air gap technique

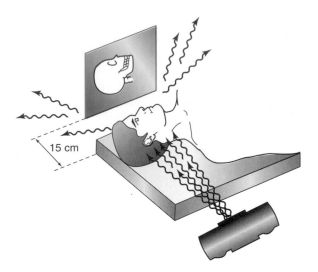

FIGURE 6-25 The air gap technique used in magnification radiography of the lateral skull.

has found some use in magnification radiography, where increased OID is already present, as well as in some institutions where chest radiography is performed with a 10 inch air gap and a 10 foot SID. It is estimated that, for a small body part (10 cm), a 10 inch air gap will clean up scatter as well as a 15:1 grid. The clean up is not as efficient for a larger body part (20 cm).[1] The air gap technique results in patient dose that is the same as, or slightly less than, using a comparable grid. Exposure may be slightly less because a grid absorbs some of the transmitted photons (grid cutoff), whereas the air gap technique does not.

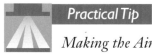

Important Relationship

Air Gap Technique and Scatter Control

The air gap technique is an alternative to using a grid to control scatter reaching the image receptor. By moving the image receptor away from the patient, more of the scatter radiation will miss the IR. The greater the gap, the less scatter reaches the IR.

Practical Tip

Making the Air Gap Technique Work

Using an increased OID is necessary for the air gap technique. However, this decreases image quality. To decrease unsharpness and increase recorded detail, the radiographer must increase SID.

---

[1]Curry TS, Dowdy JE, Murry RC: *Christensen's physics of diagnostic radiology*, ed 4, Philadelphia, 1990, Lea & Febiger.

Scatter Control and Digital Imaging

Digital imaging systems work by taking the amount of x-ray exposure reaching the image receptor and manipulating the resulting information to produce an image with appropriate density or brightness. There are certain considerations about digital systems that make scatter control even more critical than with film-screen systems.

Compared with film-screen imaging, digital imaging systems are responsive to a wider range of x-ray photons, especially the very low energy photons, such as in scatter. As with film-screen imaging, increased scatter reduces image contrast. Failure to collimate or use a grid when appropriate results in excessive scatter reaching the IR and reduces image quality.

Practical Tip

Shielding the IR when making more than one exposure

Because digital imaging systems are highly sensitive to low energy radiation, the radiographer should place lead shields over the areas not being exposed when including more than one image on the IR.

If the amount of x-ray exposure reaching the IR is low, the digital system will work to produce the appropriate density, resulting in an image with a noisy, mottled appearance. This can occur with all forms of grid cutoff or if the mAs is not increased to compensate for adding a grid or changing to a higher ratio grid. Excessive noise or mottle in a digital image is one of the primary reasons for repeating the image.

If the digital IR receives too much exposure, the system produces appropriate density, but image contrast is decreased because of excessive scatter. This may occur when a grid is removed and mAs is not decreased, or by not making adjustments in mAs when a change is made to a lower ratio grid.

Important Relationship

Digital Imaging and Scatter Control

Digital imaging systems are very sensitive to scatter radiation, as well as to overexposure and underexposure that results from grid cutoff and failure to make adjustments in mAs when needed. All of these factors result in reduced image quality.

Scatter control is important when using digital imaging systems. The important relationships throughout this chapter hold true for digital imaging and are key factors in producing optimal images. Reducing the amount of scatter produced through beam restriction, reducing the amount of scatter reaching the image receptor by using a grid, avoiding grid cutoff errors, and making appropriate exposure adjustments as needed all help to produce optimal digital images.

FILM CRITIQUE

1. Evaluate each radiograph and discuss its quality (Figures 6-26 and 6-27).
2. For each image, evaluate its exposure variables and discuss their effect on the quality of the image, regardless of whether it is apparent on the radiograph.
3. For each image, identify any adjustments that could be made in the exposure factors to produce an optimal image.

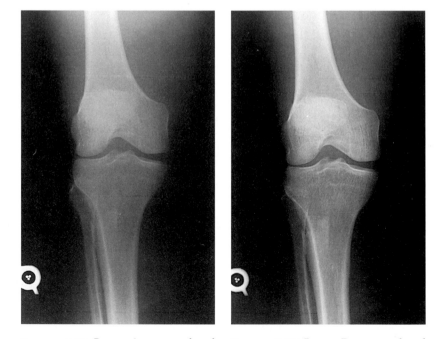

FIGURE 6-26 Image A was produced using 70 kVp, 100 mA at 0.016 s, 400 speed film-screen combination, a 40-inch source-to-image receptor distance, and no grid.

FIGURE 6-27 Image B was produced using 70 kVp, 50 mA at 0.160 s, 400 speed film-screen combination, a 40-inch source-to-image receptor distance, and a 12:1 grid ratio.

1. The projected shape of the unrestricted primary beam is
   A. square.
   B. rectangular.
   C. circular.
   D. elliptical.

2. The purpose of beam restricting devices is to _____ by changing the size and shape of the primary beam.
   A. increase patient dose
   B. decrease scatter radiation
   C. increase density
   D. decrease contrast

3. The most effective type of beam-restricting device is the
   A. cone.
   B. aperture diaphragm.
   C. cylinder.
   D. collimator.

4. Of the beam-restricting devices listed in question 3, which two are most similar to one another?
   A. A and B
   B. A and C
   C. B and C
   D. B and D

5. The purpose of automatic collimation is to ensure that
   A. the quantity of scatter production is minimal.
   B. the field size does not exceed the image receptor size.
   C. maximal recorded detail and contrast are achieved.
   D. radiographic density is maintained.

6. When making a significant increase in collimation
   A. mAs should be increased.
   B. kVp should be increased.
   C. mAs should be decreased.
   D. kVp should be decreased.

7. Which one of the following increases as collimation increases?
   A. Density
   B. Scatter production
   C. Fog
   D. Contrast

8. Which of the following is true of positive beam-limiting devices?
   A. They are required on all radiographic installations.
   B. They are required on all new radiographic installations.
   C. They have never been required on radiographic installations.
   D. They were once required on new radiographic installations.

9. The purpose of a grid in radiography is to
   A. increase density.
   B. increase contrast.
   C. decrease patient dose.
   D. increase recorded detail.

10. Grid ratio is defined as the ratio of the
   A. height of the lead strips to the distance between them.
   B. width of the lead strips to their height.
   C. number of lead strips to their width.
   D. width of the lead strips to the width of the interspace material.

11. Compared with parallel grids, focused grids
   A. have a greater grid frequency and lead content.
   B. can be used with either side facing the tube
   C. have a wider range of grid ratios and frequencies.
   D. allow more transmitted photons to reach the image receptor.

12. With which one of the following grids would a convergent line be formed if imaginary lines from its grid lines were drawn in space above it?
   A. Linear focused
   B. Crossed focused
   C. Linear parallel
   D. Crossed parallel

13. If 15 mAs is used to produce a particular level of radiographic density without a grid, what mAs would be needed to produce that same level of density using a 16:1 grid?
   A. 45
   B. 60
   C. 90
   D. 105

14. Grid cutoff, regardless of the cause, is most recognizable radiographically as reduced
   A. contrast.
   B. recorded detail.
   C. density.
   D. positioning.

15. Off-focus grid cutoff occurs by using an SID that is not
    A. within the focal range of the grid.
    B. equal to the focal distance of the grid.
    C. at the level of the convergent line of the grid.
    D. at the level of the convergent point of the grid.

16. The type of motion most used for moving grids today is
    A. longitudinal.
    B. reciprocating.
    C. circular.
    D. single stroke.

17. A grid should be used whenever the anatomic part size exceeds
    A. 3 cm
    B. 6 cm
    C. 10 cm
    D. 12 cm

18. The air gap technique uses an increased _____ instead of a grid.
    A. kVp
    B. mAs
    C. SID
    D. OID

CHAPTER 7

Image Receptors

OBJECTIVES

1 Define all of the key terms in this chapter.

2 State all of the important relationships in this chapter.

3 Describe the layers that make up radiographic film.

4 Explain how the latent image is formed.

5 Differentiate between direct-exposure film and screen film, single and double emulsion.

6 Describe film characteristics, including speed, contrast, latitude, spectral sensitivity, and crossover.

7 Describe the purpose and function of intensifying screens.

8 Describe the layers that make up intensifying screens.

9 Explain how screens can be characterized based on the type of phosphor, spectral emission, and screen speed.

10 Demonstrate use of the intensification factor (IF).

11 Demonstrate use of the mAs conversion formula for screens.

12 Describe factors that affect screen speed.

13 Explain the effect screen speed has on recorded detail.

14 Describe two major intensifying screen maintenance concerns.

15 Describe the function and construction of a cassette.

16 Describe the components of the computed radiography (CR) image receptor and explain how the latent image is created.

17 Describe the components of the direct readout digital (DR) image receptor and explain how the latent image is created.

18 Differentiate between DR systems that use direct conversion and indirect conversion.

19 Explain considerations specific to CR systems.

KEY TERMS

supercoat
emulsion
silver halide
base layer
latent image
manifest image
latent image centers
direct-exposure film
screen film
double-emulsion film
single-emulsion screen film
speed
spectral sensitivity

spectral emission
spectral matching
crossover
intensifying screen
phosphor
luminescence
fluorescence
phosphorescence
protective layer
phosphor layer
reflecting layer
absorbing layer
base

rare earth elements
screen speed
intensification factor (IF)
relative speed
mAs conversion formula for screens
quantum mottle
film-screen contact
imaging plate (IP)
flat panel direct capture detector

Double-emulsion radiographic film, as used in a cassette with intensifying screens, is the most common film-screen image receptor used in radiography today. The intensifying screens absorb the transmitted x-rays and produce light, which exposes the film. The film records the image based on the pattern of transmitted x-rays and the light produced by the intensifying screens. The cassette is the rigid, light-tight container that holds the screens and film in close contact.

The photostimulable phosphor imaging plate in a cassette, as used in computed radiography (CR), is the most common digital image receptor. The photostimulable phosphor absorbs the pattern of exit radiation. The CR cassette protects and supports the imaging plate.

Radiographic Film

Several types of radiographic film are used in medical imaging departments, depending on the specific application. Film manufacturers produce film in a variety of sizes, ranging from 20×25 cm (8×10 inches) to 35×43 cm (14×17 inches) (Figure 7-1).

FILM CONSTRUCTION

The composition of film can be described in layers (Figure 7-2). The outside layer is called the *supercoat*. The **supercoat** is a durable protective layer that is intended to prevent damage to the sensitive emulsion layer underneath it.

The next layer is the emulsion layer. The **emulsion** layer is the radiation-sensitive and light-sensitive layer of the film. The emulsion of film consists of silver halide crystals suspended in gelatin. **Silver halide** is the material that is sensitive to radiation and light. Although the precise formulations of silver halide used by

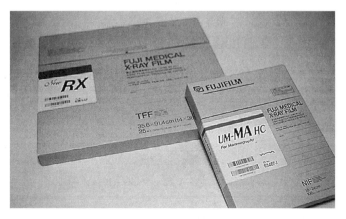

FIGURE 7-1 Radiographic film is available in a variety of types and sizes.

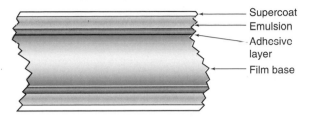

FIGURE 7-2 Composition of radiographic film.

radiographic film manufacturers are held as proprietary information, it is believed that silver bromide (AgBr) and silver iodide (AgI) make up the emulsion layer of film. In addition, it is believed that silver bromide constitutes 90% to 99% of the silver halide in film emulsions and that silver iodide makes up the remaining 1% to 10%.

A fairly recent innovation incorporated into manufacturing film is *tabular grain* (or *T-grain*) technology. Instead of using randomly shaped silver halide crystals in the emulsion layers, T-grain film uses flat silver halide crystals that can be dispersed more evenly in the emulsion layer gelatin than conventional crystals (Figure 7-3). This advancement is intended to increase the recorded detail of the radiographs produced with this film. This technology has been well accepted by the radiography industry, and T-grain film is widely used today.

The final layer of film is the base layer. The **base layer** is polyester (plastic) that gives the film physical stability. The emulsion layer is fairly fragile and must have this plastic

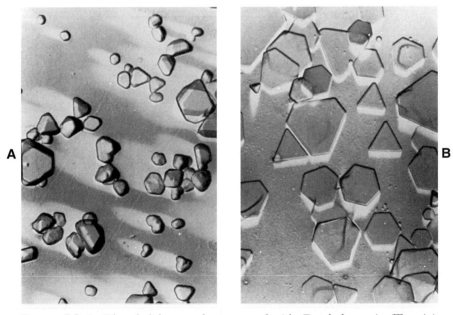

FIGURE 7-3 A, Silver halide crystals, compared with, **B,** tabular grain (T-grain) silver halide crystals.

base so that the film can be handled and processed, yet remain physically strong after processing. Most film used in radiographic procedures has a blue dye or tint added to the base layer to decrease eye strain while one views the finished radiograph.

Between the emulsion layer and the base layer is an adhesive. The adhesive simply adheres one layer of the film to another.

LATENT IMAGE FORMATION

The term **latent image** refers to that image that exists on film after that film has been exposed but before it has been processed. Radiographic film processing changes the latent image into a manifest image. The term **manifest image** refers to the image that exists on film after exposure and processing. The manifest image typically is called the *radiographic image*.

The specific way in which the latent image is formed is not really known, but the Gurney-Mott theory of latent image formation is most widely believed to be the manner in which this process happens. To explain latent image formation, it is necessary to describe what happens at the molecular level in the emulsion layer of film, specifically what happens to silver halide crystals when exposed to x-rays and light. Silver halide is made up of both silver bromide and silver iodide. However, because silver bromide (AgBr) is the primary constituent of the silver halide in the emulsion layer of film, only silver bromide is discussed. The process by which the latent image is formed is precisely the same for silver iodide as it is for silver bromide.

Latent image formation as described here is depicted in Figure 7-4. Silver (Ag) and bromide (Br) are bound together as a molecule in such a way that they share an electron (Figure 7-4, A). This electron is shared through ionic bonding because silver is a transitional atom, having only one electron in its outer shell, and it tends to either lose it or share it. The silver in AgBr is in effect an ion because it shares only its outer-shell electron with bromide. Energy in the form of x-rays or light is absorbed by the emulsion layer(s) of radiographic film. This energy absorption raises the conductivity level of the electrons in the AgBr molecules, and these electrons move faster as a result. If enough energy is absorbed by a particular AgBr molecule, the bromide will lose an electron. The silver, in effect, becomes a positive ion because it loses its shared electron to the newly ionized bromide (Figure 7-4, B, C).

Physical imperfections in the lattice or architecture of the emulsion layers occur during the film manufacturing process. These imperfections are called *sensitivity specks*. Each sensitivity speck serves as an electron trap, trapping the electrons lost by the bromide when x-ray or light exposure occurs. Therefore these sensitivity specks become negatively charged (Figure 7-4, D).

Because the sensitivity specks are negatively charged, the positive silver ions that are liberated from bromide are attracted to them (Figure 7-4, E). Every silver ion that is attracted to an electron becomes neutralized by that electron, therefore becoming metallic silver (Figure 7-4, F). The more x-ray or light exposure in a particular area of the film, the more electrons and silver available to be attracted to the sensitivity specks. The bromide liberated by x-ray or light exposure is neutral and is simply absorbed into the emulsion.

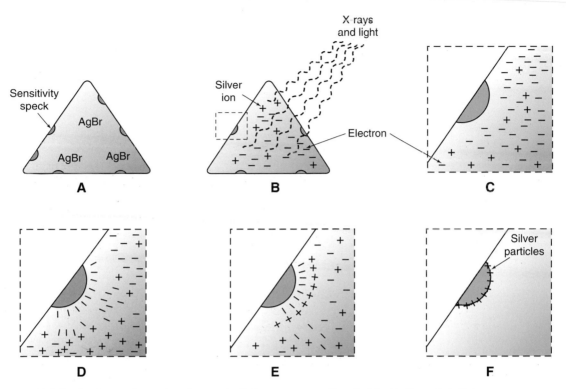

FIGURE 7-4 Latent image formation theory. **A,** Before exposure, silver halide (AgBr and AgI) is suspended in gelatin in the emulsion layer. Sensitivity specks exist as physical imperfections in the film lattice. **B,** Exposure to x-rays and light ionizes the silver halide. **C,** Negatively charged electrons and positively charged silver ions float freely in the emulsion gelatin. **D,** Sensitivity specks trap electrons. **E,** Each trapped electron attracts a silver ion. **F,** Silver clumps around the sensitivity specks.

Several sensitivity specks with many silver ions attracted to them become **latent image centers**. These latent image centers appear as radiographic density on the manifest image after processing. It is believed that for a latent image center to appear, it must contain at least three sensitivity specks that have at least three silver atoms each. The more exposure to the film, the more metallic silver that is apparent on the radiograph as radiographic density.

Important Relationship

Sensitivity Specks and Latent Image Centers

Sensitivity specks serve as the focal point for the development of latent image centers. After exposure, these specks trap the free electrons and then attract and neutralize the positive silver ions. After enough silver is neutralized, the specks become a latent image center and are converted to black metallic silver after chemical processing.

TYPES OF FILM

Two general types of film are used in diagnostic imaging: direct-exposure film and screen film. Direct-exposure film is used without intensifying screens, whereas screen film, used with intensifying screens, is available in single- or double-emulsion varieties.

Direct-Exposure Film

Direct-exposure film is often called *nonscreen film*. It is intended to be used in a cardboard holder (instead of a cassette) and without intensifying screens. It has a single emulsion that is significantly thicker than screen film and requires more development time. Compared with screen film, direct-exposure film requires considerably more exposure and may necessitate manual processing. Although still commonly used for intraoral dental radiography, direct-exposure medical film and direct-exposure radiography generally are considered outdated technologies.

Screen Film

Screen film is the most widely used radiographic film. As its name implies, it is intended to be used with one or two intensifying screens. Compared with direct-exposure film, screen film is more sensitive to light and less sensitive to x-rays. The emulsion layers are thinner than those of direct-exposure film and require less development time. Screen film, which requires less x-ray exposure, can be either manually or automatically processed and can have either a single or double emulsion coating (sometimes referred to as *duplitized*). **Double-emulsion film** has an emulsion coating on both sides of the base and a layer of supercoat over each coating (Figure 7-5, *A*). Radiographic imaging typically uses double-emulsion film with two intensifying screens.

   Single-emulsion screen film, with only one emulsion layer, is used with a single intensifying screen. It has many uses, including duplication, subtraction, computed tomography (CT), magnetic resonance imaging (MRI), sonography, nuclear medicine, mammography, and laser printing. Single-emulsion film contains an anticurl/antihalation layer, which differentiates it from double-emulsion film (Figure 7-5, *B*).

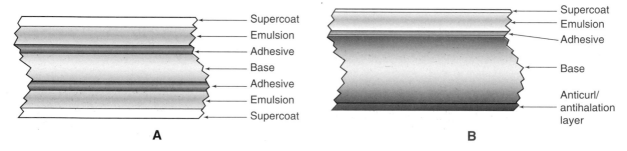

FIGURE 7-5 A, Cross-section of double-emulsion, and, **B,** single-emulsion film.

The anticurl/antihalation layer is a colored backing on single-emulsion film that prevents film from curling and prevents halation. *Halation* refers to an image being recorded on the film by reflected light that exposes the emulsion a second time. This unwanted light could come from an intensifying screen used in mammography; from the light source used in multiformat cameras in CT, MRI, nuclear medicine, or sonography; or from the light source used in radiographic duplicators and subtractors. The dull side of single-emulsion film is the emulsion side, and the shiny side is the anticurl/antihalation side. This colored backing is removed during processing.

FILM CHARACTERISTICS

Current manufacturers of medical imaging film offer a wide variety of films, which differ not only in size and general type but also in film speed, film contrast, exposure latitude, spectral sensitivity, and crossover.

Film Speed, Film Contrast, and Exposure Latitude

Film **speed** is the degree to which the emulsion is sensitive to x-rays or light. The greater the speed of a film the more sensitive it is. This increase in sensitivity results in less exposure necessary to produce a specific density. Two primary factors affect the speed of radiographic film. Both of these factors deal with the silver halide crystals that are found in the emulsion layer(s) of film. The first factor deals with the number of silver halide crystals present, and the second factor deals with the size of these silver halide crystals. Radiographic film manufacturers manipulate film speed by manipulating both of these factors in the production of specific speeds of radiographic film.

Important Relationship

Silver Halide and Film Sensitivity

As the number of silver halide crystals increases, film sensitivity or speed increases; as the size of the silver halide crystals increases, film sensitivity or speed increases.

Important Relationship

Film Speed and Radiation Exposure

The faster the speed of a film, the less radiation exposure needed to produce a specific density.

Film contrast refers to the ability of radiographic film to provide a certain level of image contrast. High-contrast film accentuates more black and white areas, whereas low-contrast film primarily shows shades of gray. Exposure latitude is closely related to film contrast.

Film speed, contrast, and latitude are graphically demonstrated in a film's characteristic (sensitometric) curve. Sensitometry is the study of the relationship between radiation exposure and the amount of density produced. This information is displayed as a curve on a graph (Figure 7-6), and every film has a different curve. Film sensitometry is discussed in greater detail in Chapter 9.

Spectral Sensitivity

Spectral sensitivity refers to the color of light to which a particular film is most sensitive. In radiography, there are generally two categories of spectral sensitivity films: blue-sensitive and green-sensitive (orthochromatic). When radiographic film is used with intensifying screens, it is important to match the spectral sensitivity of the film with the spectral emission of the screens. **Spectral emission** refers to the color of light produced by a particular intensifying screen. In radiography, two categories of spectral emission generally exist: blue light–emitting screens and green light–emitting screens. It is critical to use blue-sensitive film with blue light–emitting

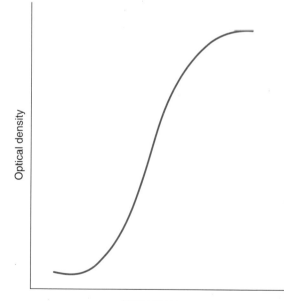

FIGURE 7-6 The characteristic (sensitometric) curve graphically represents the relationship between varying x-ray exposure and image density.

screens and green-sensitive film with green light–emitting screens. **Spectral matching** refers to correctly matching the color sensitivity of the film to the color emission of the intensifying screen. An incorrect match of film and screens based on spectral emission and sensitivity results in radiographs that display inappropriate levels of radiographic density.

Important Relationship

Spectral Matching and Density

To best use a film-screen system, the radiographer must match the color sensitivity of the film with the color emission of the intensifying screen. Failure to do so results in suboptimal density.

Spectral sensitivity also relates to the color of light produced with safelight filters. In the darkroom, safelight filters are placed in safelights to produce a particular color of light for illumination. It is important to use the appropriate safelight filter in all darkroom safelights. The filter being used is based on the spectral sensitivity of the film being handled in that darkroom. The GBX filter is safe for both blue- and green-sensitive film. GBX simply stands for green/blue x-ray. The Wratten 1A safelight filter is safe for green-sensitive film only, and the Wratten 6B safelight filter is safe for blue-sensitive film only. Most laser film has to be handled in total darkness without any darkroom illumination whatsoever because of its sensitivity to the color of light produced by safelight filters. An incorrect match between the type of safelight filter and the spectral sensitivity of film results in unusually high levels of safelight fogging on the film. This fogging appears radiographically as a film with increased density and decreased contrast.

Practical Tip

Spectral Emission and Spectral Sensitivity

The spectral emission of intensifying screens must be matched to the spectral sensitivity of the film. The spectral emission of safelight filters in the darkroom must be compatible with the spectral sensitivity of the film.

Crossover

Crossover is a problem that is unique to double-emulsion film used with intensifying screens. **Crossover** refers to light that has been produced by an intensifying screen that exposes one emulsion and then crosses over the base layer of the film to expose the other emulsion (Figure 7-7, A). Crossover is a radiographic problem because it decreases recorded detail as seen on the image.

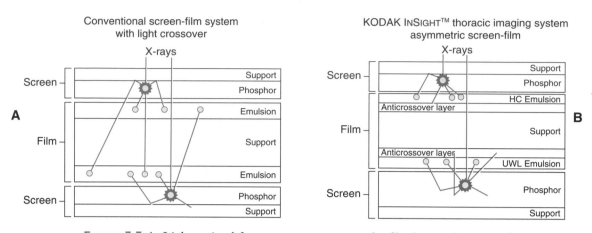

FIGURE 7-7 **A,** Light emitted from one screen crosses the film base and exposes the opposite emulsion in a conventional film-screen system. **B,** The asymmetric film-screen system has a faster back screen as well as a unique film that includes two different emulsions and zero-crossover or anticrossover technology.

Progress has been made in the reduction of crossover. The use of silver halide crystals created with T-grain technology significantly lowers crossover. In addition, another recent innovation in double-emulsion film is referred to as *zero-crossover technology.* Adding an anticrossover layer on each side of the base layer next to each emulsion layer has effectively eliminated crossover.

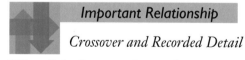

Important Relationship

Crossover and Recorded Detail

When light from one intensifying screen crosses over the film base and exposes the emulsion on the opposite side, loss of recorded detail occurs. Reducing crossover improves recorded detail.

The Kodak InSight™ Thoracic Imaging System is an example of zero-crossover technology (Figure 7-7, B). This system starts with a film with two different emulsions, one with relatively high film contrast and the other with low film contrast. This atypical film is combined with two very different intensifying screens, one much faster than the other (termed *asymmetric screens*). Zero-crossover layers ensure that the images form independently on each side of the base. The composite image produced with this system demonstrates lung detail, as well as anatomy in the area of the mediastinum.

Intensifying Screens

PURPOSE AND FUNCTION

An **intensifying screen** is a device found in radiographic cassettes that contains phosphors that convert x-ray energy into light, which then exposes the radiographic film (Figure 7-8). The **phosphor** is a chemical compound that emits visible light when struck by radiation. The purpose of intensifying screens is to decrease the patient's radiation dose when compared with use of an image receptor that does not use intensifying screens, such as direct-exposure radiography. With direct-exposure radiography, only the exit radiation produces the image of the body part. The film is placed inside a light-tight holder and then used as the image receptor. The addition of intensifying screens allows the radiographer to use significantly less mAs (the product of milliamperage and exposure time) compared with not using screens. This decreases the patient dose and allows shorter exposure times to be used. The primary trade-off or disadvantage to using intensifying screens is the reduction of recorded detail in the radiographic image.

Important Relationship

Screens, Patient Exposure, and Recorded Detail

Compared with direct-exposure radiography, adding intensifying screens reduces patient exposure but also reduces recorded detail.

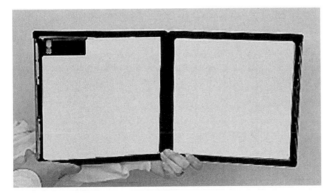

FIGURE 7-8 Typical set of intensifying screens seen inside a cassette.

From Mosby's radiographic instructional series: radiographic imaging, St Louis, 1998, Mosby.

Intensifying screens intensify or amplify the energy to which they are exposed. Without screens, the total amount of energy to which the film is exposed consists of only x-rays. With screens, the total amount of energy to which the film is exposed is divided between x-rays and light. When intensifying screens are used, approximately 90% to 99% of the total energy to which the film is exposed is light. X-rays account for the remaining 1% to 10% of the energy.

LUMINESCENCE

Intensifying screens operate by a process known as *luminescence*. **Luminescence** is the emission of light from the screen when stimulated by radiation. Intensifying screens may luminesce in two ways. The desired type of luminescence in imaging is fluorescence. **Fluorescence** refers to the ability of phosphors to emit visible light only while exposed to x-rays. *Phosphorescence* is another term to describe screen light emission. **Phosphorescence** occurs when screen phosphors continue to emit light after the x-ray exposure has stopped. Phosphorescence is sometimes called *screen lag* or *afterglow;* this result is undesirable.

SCREEN CONSTRUCTION

As with radiographic film, the construction of screens can be described in layers (Figure 7-9). The outermost layer, found closest to the film, is the protective layer. The **protective layer** is made of plastic and protects the fragile phosphor material beneath it. The **phosphor layer,** or active layer, is the most important screen component because it contains the phosphor material that absorbs the transmitted x-rays and converts them to visible light. Sometimes a light-absorbing dye is added to the phosphor layer to decrease the total amount of light striking the film.

The next layer can be either a **reflecting layer** or an **absorbing layer.** Intensifying screens usually are manufactured with one or the other, but never with both. If a reflecting layer is present, it consists of either magnesium oxide or titanium dioxide. Because phosphors emit light in all directions, their purpose is to reflect light toward the film. If an absorbing layer is used, it generally consists of a light-absorbing dye. The dye is used to absorb light directed toward it by the phosphor layer.

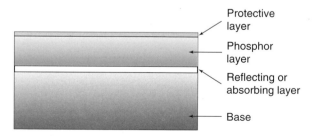

FIGURE 7-9 Cross-section of an intensifying screen.

The bottom layer of the intensifying screen, found farthest from the film, is the **base.** Made of polyester or cardboard, the base must be flexible and chemically stable. The base provides support and stability for the phosphor layer.

Intensifying screen systems used in cassettes generally include two screens. The screen that is mounted in the side of the cassette facing the x-ray tube is called the *front screen*, and the screen that is mounted in the opposite side is called the *back screen*. With two screens, the film (double emulsion) is exposed to approximately twice as much light as in a single-screen system because the film is exposed to light from both sides. Some screen systems use only a single screen and are used with single-emulsion film. When a single screen is used, it is mounted as a back screen on the side of the cassette that is opposite from the tube side.

SCREEN CHARACTERISTICS

Types of Phosphors

Many different phosphor materials are available for today's intensifying screens (Table 7-1). The most common phosphor material consists of some element from the rare earth group of elements. **Rare earth elements** are those that range in atomic number from 57 to 71 on the periodic table of the elements; they are referred to as *rare earth elements* because they are relatively difficult and expensive to extract from the earth. Rare earth phosphors have replaced calcium tungstate in the modern practice of radiography. Calcium tungstate was the mainstay phosphor used in intensifying screens until the 1970s. At that time research revealed that rare earth phosphors absorb more x-rays, convert the x-rays to visible light more efficiently, and

---

TABLE 7-1   INTENSIFYING SCREEN PHOSPHOR MATERIALS AND THEIR SPECTRAL EMISSIONS

Phosphor	Spectral Emission
Calcium tungstate ($CaWO_4$)*	Blue
Rare earth elements	
Lanthanum oxybromide (LaOBr)	Blue
Yttrium tantalate ($YTaO_4$)	Ultraviolet/blue
Gadolinium oxysulfide (Gd_2O_2S)	Green
Others	
Barium lead sulfate ($BaPbSO_4$)	Blue
Barium strontium sulfate ($BaSrSO_4$)	Blue

*No longer manufactured but may be in limited use.

result in improved recorded detail in the radiographic image compared with calcium tungstate. For these reasons, rare earth phosphors have effectively replaced calcium tungstate in today's intensifying screens.

Intensifying screen phosphors can be differentiated based on the color of visible light they emit, or their spectral emission. Calcium tungstate phosphors produce light in the blue region of the spectrum, whereas rare earth phosphors may produce green or blue light depending on the phosphor (see Table 7-1). Because film emulsion is developed to be sensitive to a specific color of light, the film and screen must be matched appropriately. As discussed earlier, *spectral matching* refers to using blue-sensitive film with blue light–emitting screens and green-sensitive (orthochromatic) film with screens that emit green light. Failure to match the screen and film results in inappropriate radiographic density.

Screen Speed

The purpose of intensifying screens is to decrease the radiation dose to the patient. Because screen phosphors can intensify the action of the x-rays by converting them to visible light, the use of screens allows the radiographer to use considerably less mAs than the amount required with direct-exposure radiography. The disadvantage of using screens is the reduction in recorded detail. Screen manufacturers produce a variety of intensifying screens, which differ in how well they intensify the action of the x-rays and therefore in their capacity to produce accurate recorded detail.

The capability of a screen to produce visible light is called **screen speed,** with a faster screen producing more light than a slower screen (given the same exposure). Screen speed can be identified in a number of ways, including the intensification factor and relative screen speed.

Important Relationship

Screen Speed and Light Emission

The faster an intensifying screen, the more light emitted for the same intensity of x-ray exposure.

The intensifying action of screens can be described by a formula called the intensification factor. This factor accurately represents the degree to which exposure factors (and patient dose) are reduced when intensifying screens are used. The **intensification factor (IF)** can be stated as follows:

$$IF = \frac{\text{Exposure required without screens}}{\text{Exposure required with screens}}$$

X   Mathematical Application

The Intensification Factor

A radiograph of a hand was produced with 100 mAs using direct exposure. A radiograph of the same hand was produced with an intensifying screen system using 4 mAs, resulting in the same density as the first image. What is the IF of the screen system?

$$IF = \frac{\text{Exposure required without screens}}{\text{Exposure required with screens}}$$

$$IF = \frac{100 \text{ mAs}}{4 \text{ mAs}}$$

$$IF = 25$$

This indicates that 25 times the exposure would be needed to produce a radiograph with comparable density if a direct-exposure system were used.

Important Relationship

Screen Speed and Patient Dose

As screen speed increases, less radiation is necessary and radiation dose to the patient decreases; as screen speed decreases, more radiation is necessary and radiation dose to the patient increases.

The ability of the screen to produce visible light, and therefore density, can also be described in terms of its **relative speed.** Relative speed results from comparing screen-film systems based on the amount of light (and density) produced for a given exposure. The amount of light produced with a par (or medium) speed calcium tungstate screen system is used as the standard for comparison and is assigned a relative speed of 100. Given the same exposure, a 200 speed system is able to produce twice as much light (and density), whereas a 400 speed system will produce four times as much light as the system using a par speed calcium tungstate screen.

Important Relationship

Screen Speed and Density

For the same exposure, as screen speed increases, density increases; as screen speed decreases, density decreases.

Screen speed and density are directly proportional. The **mAs conversion formula for screens** is a formula for the radiographer to use in determining how to compensate or adjust mAs when changing intensifying screen system speeds. This formula is stated as follows:

$$\frac{mAs_1}{mAs_2} = \frac{\text{Relative screen speed}_2}{\text{Relative screen speed}_1}$$

X *Mathematical Application*

Use of the mAs Conversion Formula for Screens

If 10 mAs was used with a 400 speed screen system to produce an optimal radiograph, what mAs would be necessary to produce a radiograph with the same density using a 100 speed screen system?

$$\frac{mAs_1}{mAs_2} = \frac{\text{Relative screen speed}_2}{\text{Relative screen speed}_1}$$

$$\frac{10\ mAs}{mAs_2} = \frac{100\ \text{relative speed}}{400\ \text{relative speed}}$$

$$mAs_2 = 40$$

When changing from a 400 speed system to a 100 speed system, one needs 4 times the mAs to maintain density. This also means that the patient receives 4 times the radiation dose.

Factors Affecting Screen Speed

Most radiology departments that use film-screen technology have at least two different speeds of intensifying screen systems. A fast system usually is available with a relative speed of about 400. A 400 speed system is a good compromise between the beneficial effect of decreasing the patient dose and the detrimental effect of decreasing the recorded detail. This system should be used for radiographic procedures of the thorax, abdomen, pelvis, skull, and facial bones (excluding the mandible and nasal bones), as well as for examinations requiring the use of a contrast medium. A slower system is usually available, and it is sometimes labeled on the outside of the cassette as "detail" or "extremity." The relative speed of this system typically is 100. This system should be used when radiographing the extremities, mandible, and nasal bones, which are studies that do not require the use of a grid. Detail or extremity screen systems are relatively slow, thereby requiring greater exposure and resulting in higher patient doses. However, the anatomic parts imaged with detail or extremity screen systems generally are small; therefore they do not require large exposures. Detail or extremity screen systems produce excellent recorded detail. The radiographer must be careful in selecting the appropriate screen system for the examination ordered.

The radiographer should select the film-screen system that balances patient exposure and recorded detail.

Several factors affect how fast or slow an intensifying screen is, including absorption efficiency, conversion efficiency, thickness of the phosphor layer, and size of the phosphor crystal. Also, the presence of a reflecting layer, an absorbing layer, or dye in the phosphor layer affects screen speed.

Differences in absorption and conversion efficiency played a large part in the switch from calcium tungstate to rare earth phosphor screens. *Absorption efficiency* refers to the screen's ability to absorb the incident x-ray photons. A rare earth phosphor screen absorbs approximately 60% of the incident photons, compared with calcium tungstate, which absorbs 30% to 40%. This means that if 100 x-ray photons were to interact with these screens, the rare earth screen would absorb about 60 photons and the calcium tungstate would absorb about 35 photons. *Conversion efficiency* describes how well the screen phosphor takes these x-ray photons and converts them to visible light. Once again, the rare earth phosphors are superior. Rare earth phosphors produce three to four times the amount of visible light per absorbed photon than does calcium tungstate. The increased absorption and conversion efficiency mean that rare earth phosphors are significantly faster than calcium tungstate. This increased speed results in the radiographer being able to substantially reduce the x-ray exposure needed to produce images with the appropriate amount of density.

Important Relationship

Rare Earth Phosphors and Speed

Rare earth phosphors are significantly faster than calcium tungstate because of increased absorption and conversion efficiency.

Because of the high absorption efficiency of rare earth phosphors, some screen manufacturers have developed cassettes that have asymmetric screens, or screens that are not identical. With asymmetric screens, the back screen is faster than the front, which compensates for the reduction of x-ray photons that were absorbed by the front screen. In this situation, having a faster back screen will equalize the light exposure to both sides of the film emulsion.

For both calcium tungstate and rare earth phosphors, the thickness of the phosphor layer and the size of the crystal also have an impact on screen speed. A thicker phosphor layer contains more phosphor material than a thinner phosphor layer. The phosphor is the material that converts x-rays into light, so if more phosphor material is present in a screen, more light will be produced, increasing the screen speed. The size of the phosphor material crystals also affects screen speed. Larger phosphor crystals produce more light than a smaller phosphor crystals. Again, more light being produced means that the screen is faster.

Important Relationship

Phosphor Thickness, Crystal Size, and Screen Speed

As the thickness of the phosphor layer increases, the speed of the intensifying screen increases; as the size of the phosphor crystals increases, the speed of the screen increases.

The final factors that affect screen speed are the presence or absence of a reflecting layer, a light-absorbing layer, or light-absorbing dyes in the phosphor layer. A reflecting layer is used to increase screen speed by reflecting light back toward the film (Figure 7-10). A light-absorbing layer or light-absorbing dyes present in the phosphor layer are used to decrease screen speed by absorbing light that would otherwise reach and expose the film.

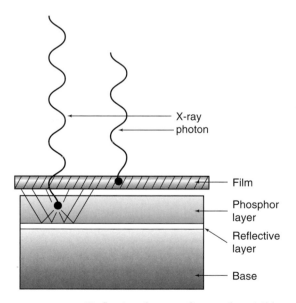

FIGURE 7-10 Reflecting layer redirects the visible light emitted by the screen phosphor toward the film emulsion. This process increases the speed of the screen but also results in a loss of recorded detail.

Screen Speed and Recorded Detail

As stated earlier, the purpose of using intensifying screens rather than direct exposure is to decrease patient dose. Screens accomplish this purpose very well but at the expense of recorded detail.

When a phosphor crystal is energized by an x-ray photon, light is emitted from the crystal and spreads out toward the film emulsion. The actual physical area of the film exposed to light from a single phosphor crystal is greater than the area of film that would be exposed by an x-ray photon (Figure 7-11). This spreading out of the radiographic information decreases the recorded detail of that image, creating more image unsharpness. Light that originates from larger crystals or farther from the film emulsion (with a thicker phosphor layer) has more spread, resulting in an even greater loss of recorded detail.

The presence or absence of a reflecting layer, an absorbing layer, or light-absorbing dyes also affects recorded detail. Because reflecting layers cause the light photons to travel farther and spread out more, screens with reflecting layers decrease recorded detail. Screens with absorbing layers or light-absorbing dyes that have been added to the phosphor layers reduce the speed of the screen and, by absorbing the lower-energy light photons, improve the level of recorded detail. The effect of these screen construction factors on screen speed, recorded detail, and patient dose are summarized in Table 7-2.

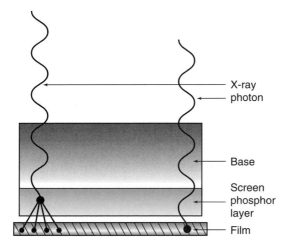

FIGURE 7-11 In comparison with the x-ray photon that directly exposes the film, the x-ray photon that interacts with the intensifying screen produces visible light. Before the film is exposed, the light spreads out, resulting in a loss of recorded detail.

TABLE 7-2   SUMMARY OF EFFECT OF SCREEN FACTORS ON SCREEN SPEED, RECORDED DETAIL, AND PATIENT DOSE

Screen Factor	Screen Speed	Recorded Detail	Patient Dose
Thicker phosphor layer	↑	↓	↓
Larger phosphor crystal size	↑	↓	↓
Reflective layer	↑	↓	↓
Absorbing layer	↓	↑	↑
Dye in phosphor layer	↓	↑	↑

Important Relationship

Screen Speed and Recorded Detail

With any given phosphor type, as screen speed increases, recorded detail decreases, and as screen speed decreases, recorded detail increases.

The type of phosphor material, either a rare earth element or calcium tungstate, affects recorded detail. Although it seems paradoxical, film-screen systems that use rare earth phosphors produce greater recorded detail than calcium tungstate systems. Because rare earth phosphors are much more efficient at absorbing the x-ray photons and converting them to light, it is possible to have a fast system with a screen that has a thin phosphor layer, small crystals, or both. It is also possible to use a slower speed film with rare earth screens to maintain an increase in relative speed, compared with calcium tungstate, and improve recorded detail. Rare earth screens have become popular because they are faster than calcium tungstate and also produce images with better recorded detail.

Quantum Mottle

Quantum mottle, commonly called *image noise*, can be defined as the statistical fluctuation in the quantity of x-ray photons that contribute to image formation per square millimeter. When a very low number of photons are needed by the intensifying screens to produce appropriate image density, the image appears mottled or splotchy. This appearance can also be described as a "salt and pepper look," versus a consistent, homogeneous density. This mottled appearance is often a direct result of using very fast speed film-screen systems that require very small amounts of exposure. Quantum mottle decreases recorded detail, which results in a radiographic image that is grainy, or noisy, in appearance (Figure 7-12, A). An optimal image displays more recorded detail (Figure 7-12, B). The only strategy for

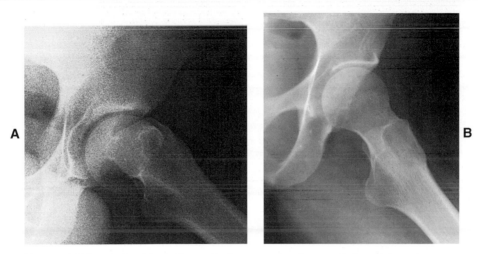

FIGURE 7-12 A, This hip radiograph demonstrates the mottled, grainy appearance associated with quantum mottle resulting from a low number of x-ray photons being used to produce the image. **B,** In comparison, an optimal hip image shows greater recorded detail.

reducing quantum mottle is the use of more mAs (more photons). This can be accomplished by using a slower speed system (requiring more mAs) or increasing the mAs while decreasing the kVp.

SCREEN MAINTENANCE

The maintenance of intensifying screens is significant because radiographic quality depends in large part on how well the screens are continuously maintained. Two important maintenance procedures should be performed on intensifying screens. One of these is regular cleaning. The outside surface of screens come into contact with the environment and with the hands of those unloading and loading cassettes, which results in the natural oils on fingers and hands being deposited on the screen surface. These oils tend to attract dust and dirt, which can build up to the point where they are actually imaged on radiographs as artifacts. Screen cleaning should be done routinely. The cleaning is accomplished with commercially available antistatic intensifying screen cleaner fluid and gauze pads.

Another important maintenance procedure is to check cassettes for film screen contact. Good **film-screen contact** exists when the screen or screens are in direct contact with the film. Poor film-screen contact greatly degrades recorded detail and is usually seen as a localized area of unsharpness somewhere on the radiographic image. Rarely is film-screen contact so poor that unsharpness can be seen across the entire radiograph. A major part of testing for film-screen contact is identifying problem cassettes.

Practical Tip

Identifying Cassettes

When it is necessary to find the specific cassette that has a problem, it can be done easily by numbering the cassettes. An excellent way to accomplish this is to write the cassette number (by use of a permanent black marker) in an out-of-the-way corner on the surface of one of the screens. That same number should be written on the outside of the cassette. The screen number will show up on images produced with that cassette, and if there is a problem, knowlegde of this number allows the radiographer to find and test the cassette in question.

The film-screen contact test is easily accomplished, but it requires a special wire mesh test tool (Figure 7-13). The wire mesh tool is placed on the cassette in question and radiographed with an appropriate technique. The resultant radiograph (Figure 7-14) is then viewed from a distance of approximately 6 feet to determine any areas of unsharpness, which would indicate poor recorded detail. Areas of poor contact will appear darker than areas of good contact because of the increased spreading out of the light photons. The film-screen contact test should be done every 6 to 12 months.

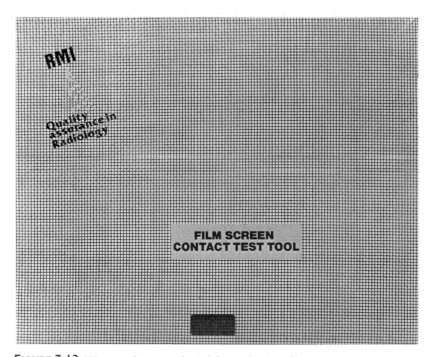

FIGURE 7-13 Wire mesh test tool used for evaluating film-screen contact.

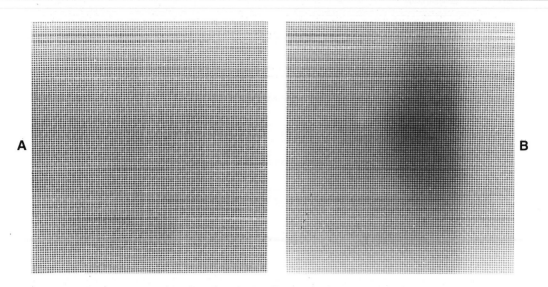

FIGURE 7-14 Images produced with wire mesh test. **A,** Proper film-screen contact. **B,** Poor film-screen contact.

From Bushong S: Radiologic science for technologists, ed 7, St Louis, 2001, Mosby.

Cassettes

The remaining component in the conventional film-screen image receptor is the cassette (Figure 7-15). Serving as a container for both the intensifying screens and the film, the cassette must be light-proof, weigh little enough to be portable, and be rigid enough not to bend under a patient's weight, all while allowing the maximum amount of radiation to pass through and reach the screens. Low x-ray–absorbing materials, such as Bakelite, magnesium, or even graphite carbon, can be found in the front of cassettes. Inside the back of cassettes may be a thin sheet of lead foil, designed to absorb backscatter before it exposes the film.

Finally, cassettes must be constructed in such a way as to maintain good film-screen contact.

Digital Imaging

Digital imaging, specifically digital radiography, involves identical x-ray production, differential absorption, and scatter control when compared with film-screen imaging. However, when the exit radiation leaves the patient, it interacts with a very different image receptor for latent image formation. The latent image is converted to digital information, which can then be manipulated by the computer.

There are two primary methods for performing digital radiography. The most common method is computed radiography (CR), using a cassette loaded with an

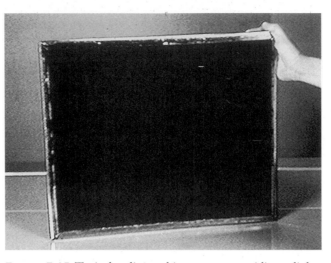

FIGURE 7-15 Typical radiographic cassette, providing a light-proof container for intensifying screens and film.

From Mosby's radiographic instructional series: radiographic imaging, St Louis, 1998, Mosby.

imaging plate containing a photostimulable phosphor (PSP). The other method of performing digital radiography is direct readout digital radiography (DR), which primarily uses a flat panel of detectors to absorb the exit radiation.

COMPUTED RADIOGRAPHY IMAGE RECEPTOR

From the outside, the image receptor used in computed radiography (CR) looks very similar to the IR for conventional film-screen radiography. Both include a cassette, which comes in a variety of sizes. The CR image receptor can be used in the same way as film-screen cassettes – in the Bucky, on the tabletop, on mobile exams. When compared with a film-screen IR that contains intensifying screens and film, an open CR cassette contains only the **imaging plate (IP)**, which looks quite similar to an intensifying screen. There is no film. As seen in Figure 7-16, the IP primarily consists of a support layer, phosphor layer, and protective layer. The key element is the phosphor layer, which consists of barium fluorohalide crystals coated with europium.

When the exit radiation interacts with the IP's phosphor layer, some energy is released as visible light (as with an intensifying screen in conventional radiography). However, the rest of the x-ray energy is absorbed and electrons (produced by a photoelectric interaction) are trapped in the phosphor layer. This constitutes the latent image.

Considerations with Computed Radiography Systems

As mentioned in Chapter 6, digital imaging systems are sensitive to a wide range of energies, including the low energy x-rays found in scatter and background radiation.

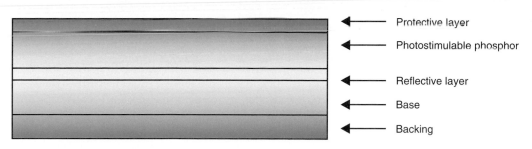

FIGURE 7-16 Cross section of CR imaging plate.

For this reason, imaging plates that are not used within 24 to 48 hours will display enough background exposure to degrade image quality.

Practical Tip

Erasure of Imaging Plates

If CR imaging plates are not used within 48 hours, they should be put through an erasure cycle before use.

The CR latent image consists of electrons trapped in the phosphor layer. This latent image will fade over time and, if the plates are not processed within a relatively short time period, the image quality will be reduced.

Practical Tip

Avoiding Fading of Latent Image

CR imaging plates should be processed within 1 hour of exposure, otherwise fading of the latent image will begin to impact image quality.

The sensitivity of a typical CR imaging plate is approximately equivalent to a 200 speed film-screen system.

Practical Tip

Adjusting the mAs for CR

When using CR, it is appropriate to adjust the mAs as if using a 200 speed film-screen system. Since many regular film-screen combinations are 400 speed, this requires doubling the mAs.

DIRECT READOUT DIGITAL RADIOGRAPHY IMAGE RECEPTOR

Direct readout digital radiography (DR) uses a **flat panel direct capture detector** array that absorbs radiation and converts the energy into electrical signals. This image receptor is different than the previously discussed IRs because it is not in a cassette but is instead in a permanent location. It may be found just below the radiographic tabletop, where you would normally find a Bucky tray, or it may be permanently configured with the x-ray tube. In either case, this IR can not be used for mobile exams.

Typically 14×17 inches in size, the DR flat panel direct capture IR consists of a large array of a combination of detectors and thin film transistors (TFTs). The exit radiation interacts with the detector and an electrical charge is created. This charge is stored temporarily in the transistor until readout. This pattern of electrical charges constitutes the latent image.

There are currently two types of detectors being manufactured, they differ in how the x-ray exposure is converted to an electric charge. The *indirect conversion* system (Figure 7-17, A) has the x-ray absorbed by a layer of cesium iodide (CsI), a scintillation phosphor, which then produces a flash of light. This light interacts with a layer of amorphous silicon (a-Si) to create the electric charge.

The *direct conversion* direct readout system (Figure 7-17, B) has the x-ray interact directly with a layer of amorphous selenium (a-Se), which then produces the electric charge. In both cases the charge is briefly stored in the thin film transistor (TFT) until readout. According to the manufacturers of these types of direct readout systems, both are very efficient at absorbing the exit radiation and quickly producing excellent quality latent image information.

Important Relationship

Latent Image Formation and Image Receptors

Latent image formation differs significantly among the three types of image receptors discussed in this chapter. Film's latent image is the result of deposits of silver ions at the sensitivity specks in the emulsion. CRs latent image is formed by electrons trapped in the barium fluorohalide crystals (in the phosphor layer). The latent image from direct readout image receptors is the electric charge stored in the transistor.

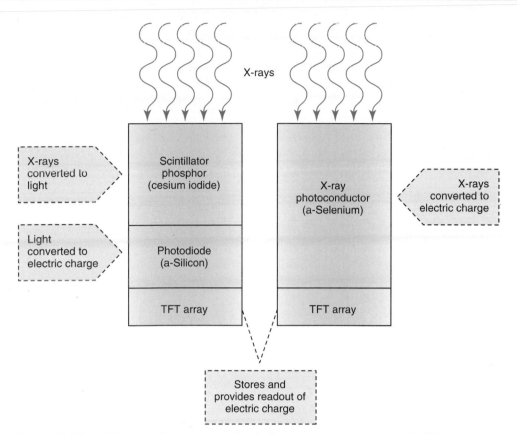

FIGURE 7-17 **A,** Direct readout system using indirect conversion process. **B,** Direct readout system using direct conversion process.

FILM CRITIQUE

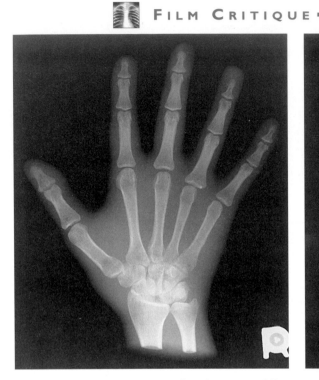

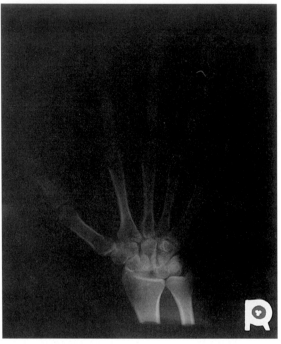

FIGURE 7-18 Image **A** was produced using 57 kVp, 50 mA at 0.040 s, 100 speed film-screen combination, and a 40-inch source-to-image receptor distance.

FIGURE 7-19 Image **B** was produced using 57 kVp, 160 mA at 0.0125 s, 400 speed film-screen combination, and a 40-inch source-to-image receptor distance.

1. Evaluate each radiograph and discuss its quality (Figures 7-18 and 7-19).
2. For each image, evaluate the exposure variables and discuss their effect on the quality of the image, regardless of whether it is apparent on the radiograph.
3. For each image, identify any adjustments that could be made in the exposure factors to produce an optimal image.

Review Questions

1. The radiation- and light-sensitive layer of radiographic film is the _____ layer.
   A. base
   B. emulsion
   C. supercoat
   D. anticurl/antihalation

2. Crossover is a radiographic problem because it decreases
   A. contrast.
   B. density.
   C. recorded detail.
   D. film speed.

3. Spectral sensitivity refers to the color sensitivity of
   A. radiographic film.
   B. safelight filters.
   C. intensifying screens.
   D. safelight filters and intensifying screens.

4. According to the Gurney-Mott theory of latent image formation, electrons liberated by radiation or light exposure are attracted to the
   A. bromide.
   B. sensitivity speck.
   C. bound silver ions.
   D. gelatin.

5. Silver halide crystals are found in the film's
   A. base.
   B. supercoat.
   C. emulsion.
   D. anticurl/antihalation layer.

6. Which of the following is the most common type of film for general radiographic examinations?
   A. Direct exposure
   B. Screen, single emulsion
   C. Screen, double emulsion
   D. Rare earth

7. Poor film-screen contact results in a loss of
   A. density.
   B. contrast.
   C. recorded detail.
   D. speed.

8. The purpose of intensifying screens is to
   A. increase radiographic density.
   B. increase recorded detail.
   C. decrease recorded detail.
   D. decrease patient dose.

9. The most common phosphor material used in today's intensifying screens is/are
   A. calcium tungstate.
   B. rare earth elements.
   C. silver halide.
   D. barium sulfate.

10. The speed of an intensifying screen can be reduced by adding
    A. more phosphor.
    B. a reflecting layer.
    C. larger phosphor crystals.
    D. dye to the phosphor layer.

11. What is the intensification factor for screens that require 5 mAs to produce the same density as produced by direct exposure using 150 mAs?
    A. 5
    B. 30
    C. 50
    D. 300

12. If 25 mAs is used with a 500 speed film-screen system to produce an optimal image, how much mAs is needed to produce the same density with 100 speed system?
    A. 5 mAs
    B. 100 mAs
    C. 125 mAs
    D. 300 mAs

13. Typically, as screen speed decreases, _____ decreases.
    A. density
    B. recorded detail
    C. patient dose
    D. x-ray exposure

14. Which of the following strategies reduces quantum mottle?
    A. Using a faster speed film-screen system
    B. Increasing kVp and reducing mAs
    C. Reducing kVp and increasing mAs
    D. Reducing kVp and reducing mAs

15. The wire mesh test tool is used to evaluate
    A. screen speed.
    B. screen resolution.
    C. screen cleanliness.
    D. film-screen contact.

16. The image receptor for computed radiography (CR) is composed of
    A. amorphous selenium.
    B. amorphous silicon.
    C. silver bromide.
    D. barium fluorohalide.

17. Both types of direct readout flat panel detector digital imaging systems convert x-ray energy into
    A. electric charges.
    B. black metallic silver.
    C. chemical energy.
    D. light energy.

18. The latent image that consists of electrons trapped in the phosphor layer is found with
    A. direct conversion direct readout digital systems.
    B. indirect conversion direct readout digital systems.
    C. film-screen radiography.
    D. CR.

19. Exposed CR imaging plates should be processed within _____ hour(s) to avoid any loss of image quality because of fading.
    A. 1
    B. 5
    C. 24
    D. 48

20. Thin film transistors (TFTs) are used in direct readout DR systems to
    A. produce a flash of light.
    B. convert the x-ray energy to an electric charge.
    C. temporarily store the electric charge.
    D. trap the electrons in the photostimulable phosphor layer.

CHAPTER 8

Radiographic Film Processing

1 Define all of the key terms in this chapter.

2 State all of the important relationships in this chapter.

3 State the purpose of radiographic processing.

4 Describe the various processing stages, systems, and rollers.

5 List the developing and fixing solution agents and state their function.

6 Discuss the role of developer temperature in processing.

7 Describe the washing and drying processing stages.

8 List problems of inadequate processing and their radiographic presentation.

9 State the importance of replenishment during processing.

10 List important considerations in the handling and storage of film before and after processing.

11 Describe the importance of darkroom design.

12 State the importance of and process of silver recovery.

13 Recognize radiographic artifacts and their causes.

KEY TERMS

latent image
manifest image
automatic processor
processing cycle
processor capacity
developing or reducing agents
superadditivity
accelerator/activator agent
restrainer
preservative (developer)
hardener (developer)
solvent
fixing agent
acidifier
preservative (fixer)
hardener (fixer)
diffusion

feed tray
entrance roller assembly
transport rollers
turnaround roller
crossover roller
guide plates
standby control
replenishment
aerial oxidation
use oxidation
flood replenishment
recirculation system
immersion heater
FIFO
silver recovery
artifact

Processing converts the invisible image on exposed film into a permanent visible radiographic image. Automatic processing equipment consists of a series of tanks, rollers, systems, and processing stages. The stages of development and fixation use a combination of chemicals that interact with the film emulsion(s) to produce the visible image.

Considerations in film handling, darkroom design, and silver recovery are also important to the overall quality of radiographs and environmental health. In addition, the prevention of radiographic artifacts is necessary for the overall production of a quality radiograph.

Because processing of digital images is significantly different from processing radiographic film, the following discussion is only applicable with radiographic film. Processing of digital images will be discussed in Chapter 12.

Purpose

The purpose of radiographic processing is to convert the latent image into a manifest image. The **latent image** is the image that exists on the film after exposure but before processing (refer to Chapter 7). The **manifest image** is the image that exists on the film after processing.

The electrochemical process that occurs according to the Gurney-Mott theory is the first step toward creating a visible image on radiographic film. Exposure of the silver bromide crystal in the film emulsion by light or x-ray photons initiates an electrochemical process. Chemical processing of the exposed film completes the conversion process and transforms the image into a permanent visible image.

Automatic Processing Equipment

An **automatic processor** (Figure 8-1) is a device that encompasses chemical tanks, a roller transport system, and a dryer system for the processing of radiographic film. Many manufacturers produce automatic processors and various models of this type of equipment. Different models of automatic processors vary in terms of processing cycle and processor capacity. **Processing cycle** refers to the amount of time it takes to process a single piece of film. This amount of time varies between 45 seconds and 3.5 minutes, depending on the processor that is used. **Processor capacity** refers to the number of films that can be processed per hour. Processor capacity depends on the film size and can be expressed in terms of the number of films of equal size processed in 1 hour, or it can be expressed in terms of the number of films of multiple sizes processed in 1 hour. Knowing the processing cycle and capacity of a processor is important when purchasing one.

The processing of a radiograph occurs in four stages: developing, fixing, washing, and drying. Each stage has its specific function and processing method.

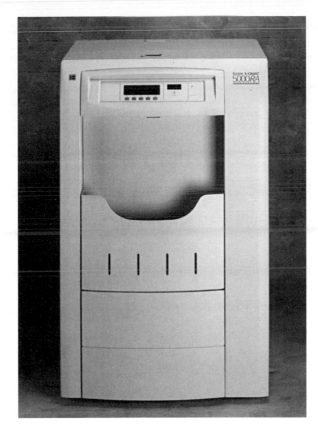

FIGURE 8-1 A type of automatic processor used in radiography.
Courtesy Eastman Kodak Company.

Processing Stages

DEVELOPING

The primary function of developing is to convert the latent image into a manifest or visible image. There are also two secondary purposes of developing. One is to amplify the amount of metallic silver on the film by increasing the number of silver atoms in each latent image center. The other is to reduce the exposed silver halide crystals into metallic silver.

During the development process, developer solution donates additional electrons to the sensitivity specks, or electron traps, in the emulsion layer(s) of the film. These additional electrons attract more silver to these areas, thereby amplifying the amount of atomic silver at each latent image center. Exposed silver halide is reduced to metallic silver when bromide and iodide ions are removed from the emulsion. The atomic silver that was exposed to radiant energy (light and x-rays) is converted to metallic silver and presented as radiographic densities. Unexposed silver halide will not react immediately to developer because it has not been ionized and will not accept electrons from the developer. Given extended exposure to developing solution or exposure to excessively heated developing solution, however, even unexposed areas of film can react to developing solution. Exposed silver halide reacts to developer by accepting electrons because neutral atomic silver that was previously bonded to either bromide or iodide has room to accept electrons in its outermost electron shell (the O-shell).

Developing or Reducing Agents

The purpose of the **developing** or **reducing agents** is to reduce exposed silver halide to metallic silver and to add electrons to exposed silver halide. Two chemicals are used to accomplish this purpose: phenidone and hydroquinone. Phenidone is said to be a fast reducer, producing gray (lower) densities. Hydroquinone is said to be a slow reducer, producing black (higher) densities.

Important Relationship

Producing Radiographic Densities

The developing agents are responsible for reducing the exposed silver halide crystals to metallic silver, visualized as optical densities. Phenidone is responsible for creating the lower densities, and hydroquinone is responsible for creating the higher densities. Their combined effect results in the range of visible densities on the radiograph.

Both phenidone and hydroquinone also act to soften and swell the emulsion(s). Phenidone and hydroquinone are said to be synergistic, or to have superadditivity. **Superadditivity** means that together these chemicals produce a greater effect on the film than they would individually. This is used to advantage by using both chemicals in combination to develop or reduce the exposed silver halide.

Accelerator or Activator Agent

The purpose of the **accelerator** or **activator agent** (sometimes also called a *buffering agent*) is to elevate and maintain the pH of the developer solution. The pH measures the alkalinity of the solution that is needed for the reducing agents. A loss of pH means a loss of developer activity. A carbonate, such as sodium carbonate, is the chemical used as this agent.

Restrainer

The purpose of the **restrainer** is to decrease the reduction or development of unexposed silver halide. Such reduction or development is generally referred to as *chemical fog* because some chemicals (usually the reducing agents) can create densities in areas of the film where no densities should be present. A bromide, such as potassium bromide, is the chemical used as this agent.

Preservative

The purpose of the **preservative** is to decrease oxidation of the developer solution. Oxidation acts to decrease the chemical activity of developer that begins almost immediately after the developer solution is mixed. A sulfite, such as sodium sulfite, is the chemical used as this agent.

Hardener

The purpose of the **hardener** is to harden the emulsion that was softened by the reducing or developing agents. This hardening process protects the radiographic image present on the film from being damaged by the roller transport system. Glutaraldehyde is the chemical used as the hardener.

Solvent

The purpose of the **solvent** is to dilute the chemicals in the developer solution, which causes these chemicals to function at their desired level of activity. The solvent is water. Developer chemicals are available in liquid form and generally are packaged in three separate packages for mixing with water.

Each of these agents and their chemicals and functions are summarized in Table 8-1.

TABLE 8-1   DEVELOPER SOLUTION AGENTS, CHEMICALS, AND THEIR FUNCTIONS

Agent	Chemical(s)	Function
Developing or reducing agents	Phenidone	Fast-reducing, produces gray densities
	Hydroquinone	Slow-reducing, produces black densities
Accelerator or activator	Sodium carbonate	Elevates and maintains solution pH
Restrainer	Potassium bromide	Decreases reduction of unexposed silver halide
Preservative	Sodium sulfite	Decreases oxidation of solution
Hardener	Glutaraldehyde	Hardens the emulsion(s)
Solvent	Water	Dilutes the chemicals

FIXING

The primary functions of the fixing stage are to remove unexposed silver halide from the film and to make the remaining image permanent. There are also two secondary functions of fixing. One is to stop the development process; the other is to further harden the emulsion(s). Fixing solution must function to remove all undeveloped silver halide while not affecting the metallic silver image.

Fixing Agent

The purpose of the **fixing agent** is to clear undeveloped silver halide from the film. A thiosulfate (sometimes also called *hypo*), such as ammonium thiosulfate, is the chemical used as this agent.

Important Relationship

Clearing the Unexposed Crystals

The fixing agent, ammonium thiosulfate, is responsible for removing the unexposed crystals from the emulsion.

Acidifier

The purpose of the **acidifier** (sometimes called a *buffer*) is to stop the development process and create an acid pH environment for the fixing agent. An acid, such as acetic acid, is the chemical used as this agent.

Preservative

The purposes of the **preservative** are to protect the fixing agent from oxidation and to maintain its activity level. Oxidization and developer carryover can decrease the strength of the fixing agent. A sulfite, such as sodium sulfite, is the chemical used as this agent.

Hardener

The purpose of the **hardener** is to further harden the emulsion to make the resultant manifest image permanent for handling. An aluminum salt, such as chrome alum, potassium alum, aluminum sulfate, or aluminum chloride, is the chemical used as this agent.

Solvent

The purpose of the solvent is to dilute the chemicals in the fixer solution so that the chemicals can function at their desired level of activity. The solvent is water. Fixer chemicals are available in liquid form and generally are packaged in two separate packages for mixing with water.

Each of these agents and their chemicals and functions are summarized in Table 8-2.

WASHING

The purpose of the washing process is to remove fixing solution from the surface of the film. This is a further step in making the manifest image permanent. If not properly washed, the resulting radiograph will show a brown staining of the image, resulting in image loss and a decrease in its diagnostic value. This staining is caused by thiosulfate (fixing agent) that remains in the emulsion(s). Some thiosulfate will always remain within the film, but the goal of washing is to remove enough so that the radiograph can be used for an extended period.

Important Relationship

Archival Quality of Radiographs

Maintaining the archival (long-term) quality of radiographs requires that most of the fixing agent be removed (washed) from the film. Staining or fading of the permanent image results when too much thiosulfate remains on the film.

TABLE 8-2   FIXER SOLUTION AGENTS, CHEMICALS, AND THEIR FUNCTIONS

Agent	Chemical(s)	Function
Fixing agent	Ammonium thiosulfate	Clears away unexposed silver halide
Acidifier	Acetic acid	Stops development
Preservative	Sodium sulfite	Prevents reaction between fixing agent and acidifier
Hardener	Chrome alum, potassium aluminum sulfate, or aluminum chloride	Hardens the emulsion
Solvent	Water	Dilutes the chemicals

The process by which washing works is referred to as *diffusion*. **Diffusion** exposes the film to water that contains less thiosulfate than the film does. Because the film contains more fixing agent than the water, the fixing agent diffuses into the water.

Eventually, thiosulfate concentrations in the wash water can become greater than those in the films that are being processed; therefore the wash water must be replaced frequently. The wash tank does not use the same replenishment system as the developer and fixer tanks. Instead, water flows freely from the input water supply through the wash tank and down the drain while the roller transport system is operating. This type of system provides a constant supply of fresh wash water to aid in the diffusion process. The moving water also causes agitation and increases diffusion.

DRYING

The final process in automatic processing is drying. The purpose of drying films is to remove 85% to 90% of the moisture from the film so that it can be handled easily and stored while maintaining the quality of the diagnostic image. As a result, finished radiographs should retain 10% to 15% of their moisture when processing is complete. If films are dried excessively, emulsion(s) can crack, which decreases the diagnostic quality of the radiograph.

Important Relationship

Archival Quality of Radiographs

Permanent radiographs must retain moisture of 10% to 15% to maintain archival quality. Excessive drying can cause the emulsion(s) to crack.

Increased relative humidity decreases the efficiency of dryers in processors, so an increased drying temperature is necessary. Processors are equipped with thermostatic controls to allow a wide range of dryer temperatures to be selected. For this chemical process to occur, specialized equipment and systems must perform concurrently to move the film through the processing stages according to the manufacturer's specifications.

Processing Systems

TANKS

An automatic processor has three tanks: one for developer solution, one for fixer solution, and a wash tank for water. These tanks are made of stainless steel to prevent corrosion, and they provide a surface that is cleaned easily. The developer tank is the deepest, followed by the fixer tank, and then the wash tank. Considering that a film moves through the processor at a constant speed, it spends most of the time in the developer tank, somewhat less time in the fixer tank, and the least time in the wash tank.

VERTICAL TRANSPORT SYSTEM

Automatic processors use a vertical transport system of rollers that advance the film through the various stages of film processing (Figure 8-2). All rollers in a processor move at the same speed. A film is introduced into the processor on the feed tray (Figure 8-3). The **feed tray** is a flat metal surface with an edge on either side that permits the film to enter the processor easily and correctly aligned. As the film enters the processor from the feed tray, the first roller assembly that it encounters is the entrance roller assembly. The **entrance roller assembly** consists of rollers that are covered with corrugated rubber (Figure 8-4). These corrugations assist in straightening out the path of the film so that it moves through the processor efficiently. Once a piece of film has moved through the roller assembly, an audible signal is given as an indication that it is safe to insert another piece of film into the processor. Ignoring this signal and inserting a piece of film too soon will cause the films to overlap. Overlapping films can cause the transport roller system to jam or cause inadequate processing of both films.

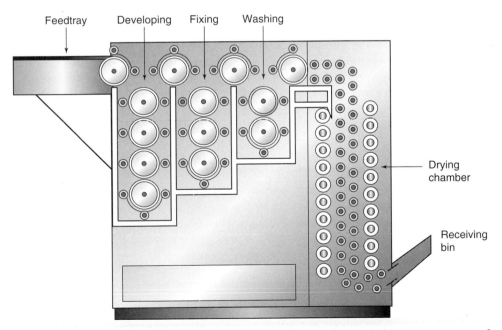

FIGURE 8-2 Cross-section of an automatic processor showing the vertical transport system of rollers.

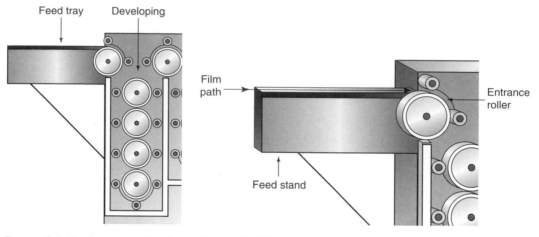

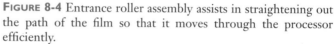

FIGURE 8-3 Feed tray permits the film to enter the processor easily and correctly aligned.

FIGURE 8-4 Entrance roller assembly assists in straightening out the path of the film so that it moves through the processor efficiently.

The next type of roller that the film encounters is a transport roller (Figure 8-5). **Transport rollers** move the film through the chemical tanks and dryer assembly. Transport rollers are found on each side of a roller assembly. As the film enters a transport assembly, the transport rollers move the film down into the tank. The rollers also move the film up through the tank on the other side of the roller assembly. A **turnaround roller** at the bottom of the roller assembly turns the film from moving down the transport assembly to moving up the assembly. Transport rollers and turnaround rollers are often called *deep rollers* because they are immersed in liquid in the processor tanks.

The final type of roller used in the vertical transport system is the crossover roller (see Figure 8-6). There are crossover assemblies between each transport assembly in the processor. The **crossover roller** assembly moves the film from one tank to another and into the dryer assembly (i.e., crossover rollers "cross" the film from one transport assembly to another). The space between the crossover rollers is typically tight, which allows the rollers to act like a squeegee on the film as it passes through the rollers. This squeegee effect assists in removing as much liquid as possible from the film before the film enters the next stage of processing. Removal of liquid makes the next stage of processing more efficient.

In addition to the different roller assemblies that make up the vertical transport system, there are also guide plates on the roller assemblies. **Guide plates** are slightly curved metal plates that properly guide the leading edge of the moving film through the roller assembly. Guide plates are located in several areas of the roller assemblies (Figure 8-7).

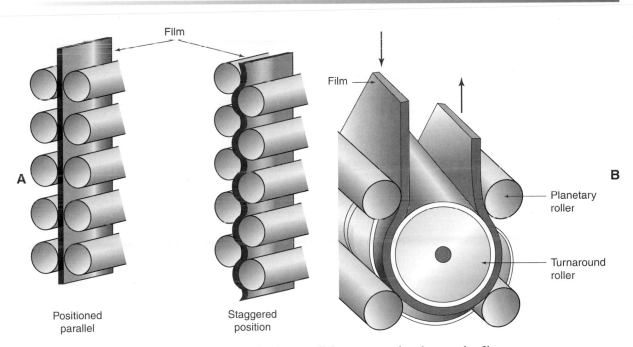

FIGURE 8-5 A, Transport rollers are positioned either parallel or staggered and move the film through the various stages of processing. **B,** Turnaround rollers at the bottom of the assembly turn the film from moving down to moving up.

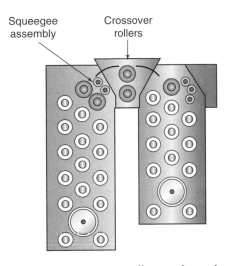

FIGURE 8-6 Crossover rollers are located between each transport assembly in the processor.

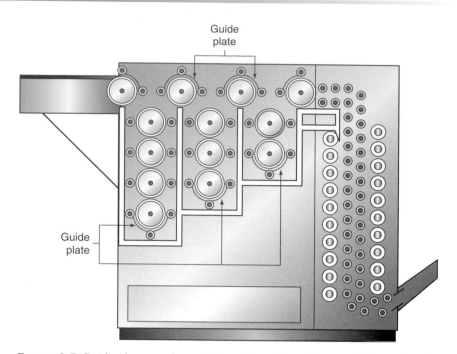

FIGURE 8-7 Guide plates are located throughout the roller assemblies and guide the leading edge of the moving film.

MOTOR DRIVE

An electric motor provides power for the roller assemblies to transport the film through the processor. The on/off switch that provides electrical power to the processor activates this motor. Most processors are also equipped with a standby control. The **standby control** is an electric circuit that shuts off power to the roller assemblies when the processor is not being used. Some wash water systems are also connected to the standby control. Pushing the standby control switch when one is ready to process a film can reactivate the roller assemblies and water intake. Typically, a timer on the standby control activates the standby circuit several minutes after the last film has been processed to stop the rollers and the circulating wash water. The purpose of this type of control is to improve cost-efficiency. Stopping the rollers when processing is not occurring reduces the wear and tear on these assemblies. Use of a standby control can also decrease water use. In addition, the standby control periodically reactivates the processor to keep chemicals mixed and temperatures stable throughout the tanks.

REPLENISHMENT SYSTEM

Replenishment refers to the replacement of fresh chemicals after the loss of chemicals during processing, specifically developer solution and fixer solution. The replenishment of chemicals used in the automatic processor is necessary because these chemicals eventually become exhausted and their ability to perform their functions decreases. Developer solution becomes exhausted through both aerial oxidation and use oxidation.

Important Relationship

Replenishment and Solution Performance

The replenishment system provides fresh chemicals to the developing and fixing solutions to maintain their chemical activity and volume when they become depleted during processing.

Aerial oxidation refers to a reduction in chemical strength as a result of exposure to air. **Use oxidation** refers to a reduction in chemical strength as a result of exposure to increased temperature over an extended period. Fixer solution becomes exhausted for several reasons: it becomes weakened from use, as a result of accumulations of silver halide that are removed from the film during the fixing process, and because developer solution remains in the film, which decreases the strength and activity of the fixer solution. Two different types of replenishment systems are available. Many processors are equipped with the ability to use both types. One type of replenishment system bases the amount of solution to be replenished on the size of the film to be processed. This type of system uses microswitches that are connected to the entrance roller assembly (Figure 8-8). These micro switches are wired to two replenishment pumps, one for developer solution and one for fixer solution. As long as a piece of film is in the entrance roller assembly, the microswitches and replenishment pumps are activated. When the replenishment pumps are activated, they pump fresh solution from a reservoir into the chemical tanks of the processor.

The volume of replenishment solution that is pumped into the chemical tanks is the same as the volume of used solution that is drained out of the processor. The amount of solution that is replenished is preset, although it can be adjusted, and depends on film size. For example, a film measuring 8×10 inches requires a lower volume of solutions than a film measuring 10×12 inches because of the difference in the physical area of both films. However, if an 8×10-inch film is run into the processor lengthwise and a 10×12-inch film is run in crosswise (Figure 8-9), the same volume of replenishment solutions will be pumped into the processor. This occurs because the microswitch system that is hooked up to the entrance roller assembly senses the film while it is in the entrance roller assembly. The dimensions of the piece of film and how it is run into the processor determine the amount of time the replenishment pumps are activated. The running length of the film (Figure 8-10) determines how long the film will be in the entrance roller assembly and therefore the volume of replenishment solutions that will be pumped into the processor. It is important to run films into the processor in a particular orientation based on film size to avoid overreplenishment or underreplenishment of solutions.

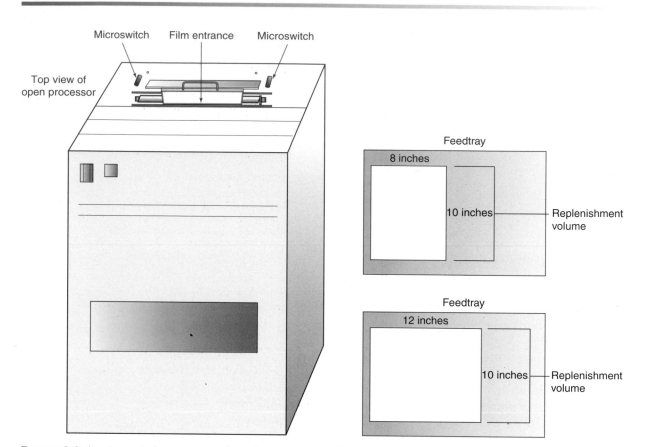

FIGURE 8-8 A microswitch is connected to the entrance roller assembly and activates the replenishment pumps while the film is in the entrance roller assembly.

FIGURE 8-9 Volume of replenishment pumped into the processor is affected by the film dimension and its orientation on the feed tray.

Practical Tip

Film Orientation for Proper Replenishment

The radiographer should align the radiographic film so that the film is horizontally placed on the feed tray and its leading edge is long. When processing two 8 × 10-inch films, the radiographer should place both films parallel to each other so that the leading edges are short.

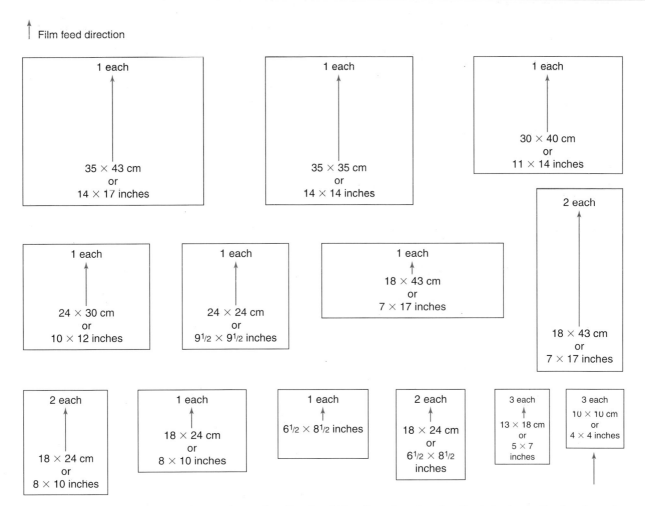

↑ Film feed direction

FIGURE 3-10 Radiographic film should be aligned so that the film is horizontally placed on the feed tray and its leading edge is long.

Overreplenishment of developer solution causes an increase in radiographic density and a decrease in radiographic contrast. Overreplenishment of fixer solution has no effect on radiographic quality but unnecessarily wastes solution. Underreplenishment of developer and fixer may cause films to jam in the roller transport system because of inadequate hardening of the film emulsion(s). Underreplenishment of developer can cause decreased density, whereas underreplenishment of fixer could result in poor archival quality of finished radiographs. Replenishment systems usually are adjusted so that more fixer solution is replenished per film in comparison to developer solution.

The second type of replenishment is called *flood replenishment*. **Flood replenishment** refers to the replenishment of solutions that occur at timed intervals, independent of the size or number of films processed. With flood replenishment, solutions are pumped into the processor every several minutes while the motor drive of the processor is on standby. The timing of the intervals is adjustable. Flood replenishment is useful in processors that process a low to medium volume of films, especially single-emulsion films. In processors that are used in this manner, the stability of developer solution and radiographic density is difficult to maintain. Developer replenisher that contains starter solution is used in conjunction with flood replenishment to maintain developer solution activity and to produce more consistent levels of density on finished radiographs.

RECIRCULATION SYSTEM

Automatic processors have a recirculation system for the developer and fixer tanks. Each tank has a separate system that consists of a pump and connecting tubing. The **recirculation system** acts to circulate the solutions in each of these tanks by pumping solution out of one portion of the tank and returning it to a different location within the same tank from which it was removed (Figure 8-11). The recirculation system keeps the chemicals mixed, which helps maintain solution activity and provides agitation of the chemicals about the film to facilitate fast processing.

Important Relationship

Recirculation and Solution Performance

Recirculation of the developer and fixer solutions is necessary to maintain solution activity and the required agitation.

Recirculation also helps maintain the proper temperature of the developer solution. The developer recirculation system includes an in-line filter that removes impurities as the developer solution is being recirculated (Figure 8-12).

Fixer orifice

Developer orifice

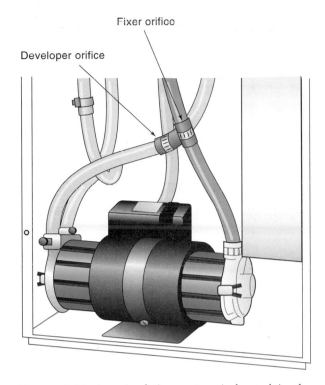

FIGURE 8-11 A recirculation system is located in the developer and fixer tanks to maintain solution activity and to provide the necessary agitation.

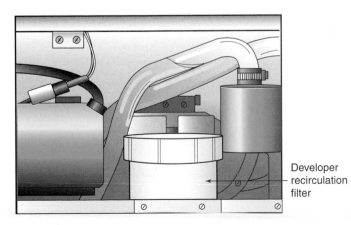

Developer recirculation filter

FIGURE 8-12 The developer recirculation filter removes impurities as the developer solution is being recirculated.

TEMPERATURE CONTROL

Temperature control of the developer solution is important because the activity of this solution depends directly on its temperature. An increase or decrease in developer temperature can adversely affect the quality of the radiographic image.

Important Relationship

Developer Temperature and Radiographic Quality

Variations in developer temperature adversely affect the quality of the radiographic image. Increasing developer temperature increases the density, and decreasing developer temperature decreases the density. Radiographic contrast also may be adversely affected by changes in the developer temperature.

In most 90-second automatic processors, developer temperature must be maintained at 93° to 95° F (33.8° to 35° C). In older processors a mixing valve connected to the water input of the processor is used to mix hot and cold water to achieve the proper temperature of water entering the processor. This water is circulated around the developer tank in water jackets to raise and maintain the temperature of the developer solution. In newer processor models an immersion heater (Figure 8-13) is used. An **immersion heater** is a heating coil that is immersed in the bottom of the developer and fixer tank. It is thermostatically controlled to heat the developer solution to its proper temperature and maintain that temperature as long as the processor is turned on. Processors that use an immersion heater are sometimes called *cold-water processors* because they can adequately use a cold-water supply and do not depend on heated water for the heating of the developer solution. Developer temperature is usually displayed on the outside of the processor (Figure 8-14). Another possible way of controlling the temperature of the developer solution is by using an in-line heat exchanger that is connected to the developer recirculation system. As developer solution is recirculated, it passes through the thermostatically controlled heat exchanger and is heated to proper temperature.

Heating
coils

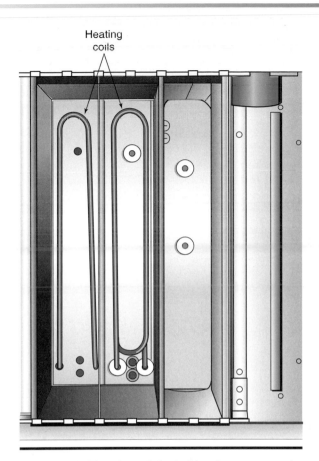

FIGURE 8-13 Top view of the inside of processor tanks. The immersion heater coil at the bottom of the developer and fixer tank heats and maintains the developer temperature.

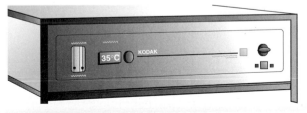

FIGURE 8-14 Developer temperature display.

DRYING SYSTEM

Radiographs must be properly dried to be viewed and stored. There are several means by which this may occur. The crossover roller assembly between the wash tank and the dryer contains several sets of squeegee rollers that remove moisture from the film.

When large 90-second processors are used, the film is further dried by hot air that is blown onto both surfaces of the film as it moves through the dryer. This air is forced through the dryer by a blower and is directed onto the film by air tubes. The temperature of the air that is used to dry films is thermostatically monitored to accurately control moisture removal from the film (Figure 8-15). Some processors, especially slower and smaller tabletop models, may use infrared lamps instead of heated air to dry films.

Important Relationship

Moisture and Archival Quality

The dryer assembly controls the amount of moisture removal to maintain the archival quality of radiographic film.

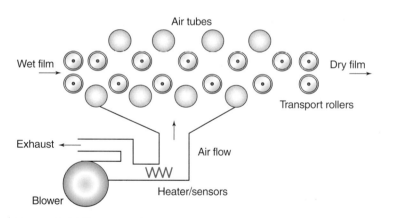

FIGURE 8-15 Processor dryer system.

Inadequate Processing

Inadequate processing is evidenced by certain appearances of the finished radiograph. Particular problems can be pinpointed by analyzing of the radiographs. These problems and the radiographic appearances that indicate them are summarized in Table 8-3.

TABLE 8-3   INDICATORS OF INADEQUATE PROCESSING

Radiographic Appearance	Processing Problem
Decrease in density	Developer exhausted Developer underreplenishment Processor running too fast Low developer temperature Developer improperly mixed
Increase in density	Developer overreplenishment High developer temperature Light leak in processor Developer improperly mixed
Pinkish stain (dichroic fog)	Contamination of developer by fixer Developer or fixer underreplenishment
Brown stain (thiosulfate stain)	Inadequate washing
Emulsion removed by developer	Insufficient hardener in developer
Milky appearance	Fixer exhausted Inadequate washing
Streaks	Dirty processor rollers Inadequate washing Inadequate drying
Water spots	Inadequate drying
Minus-density scratches	Scratches from guide plates caused by roller or plate misalignment

Film-Handling Areas

Film-handling areas in a radiology department include areas where unexposed film is stored, areas where radiographs are stored, and the processing area. Some important factors must be considered in these areas to optimize radiographic quality.

STORING UNEXPOSED FILM

Unexposed film should be stored in its original packaging so that important information about the film can be maintained. Box 8-1 presents information that is contained on the outside of film boxes.

Film boxes should be stored vertically, not horizontally, to prevent pressure artifacts on the film. Film should be stored at temperatures ranging from 50° to 70° F

Box 8-1 *Information Found on the Outside of Radiographic Film Boxes*

Brand name   Number of sheets
Expiration date   Safelight requirements
Lot number   Size
Manufacturer

Box 8-2 *Possible Consequences of Storing Unexposed Film in Environments with Improper Temperature and Relative Humidity*

Storage Environment Problem	Possible Consequence
Temperature too high	Increased fog levels
Temperature too low	Increased static discharge
Humidity too high	Increased fog levels
Humidity too low	Increased static discharge

(10° to 21° C) and a relative humidity of 40% to 60%. Film should be stored away from heat sources and ionizing radiation. Both heat and radiation can cause the silver halide in film emulsion to break down, which results in fogged film (Box 8-2). The shelf life of film, as expressed by its expiration date, must be observed. Film should not be used beyond this date. A FIFO system of rotation should be used to ensure that stored film is rotated properly into the film bin for immediate use. **FIFO** is an acronym for first in/first out. This system requires that film received first be the film that is first rotated into the working film supply. In contrast, a LIFO (last in/first out) system ensures that only the freshest film is used, while allowing older film to go to waste as it passes its expiration date.

STORING RADIOGRAPHS

To ensure the stability of film emulsions, the radiographer should make certain that a specific temperature and relative humidity range is maintained when finished radiographs are stored. Recommended ranges are between 60° and 80° F (16° to 26° C) and between 30% and 50% relative humidity. Although radiographic film generally has a "safety" designation that indicates it is nonflammable, the paper file folders that films are stored in are flammable. The area in which radiographs are stored should be designated a no-smoking area, and the radiographs should be stored on metal shelving as opposed to wood shelving to further decrease the fire hazard.

Because the space needs for the storage of radiographs are considerable, many radiology departments use remote storage sites, either on site at their respective facilities or off-site, for the long-term storage of radiographs. The miniaturization of radiographs in the form of microfilm, microfiche, or 35-mm film has also become popular. Storing images digitally on computer disks or tape is becoming increasingly popular and will likely continue to rise in popularity.

The need for security of stored radiographs is also an important consideration. Radiographs are legally considered part of the patient's medical records, which gives ownership of and responsibility for those records to the institution that produced them. Access to radiographs must be well controlled. Many facilities are finding it advantageous to not release original radiographs to requesting parties but instead to release duplicated copies of radiographs. This ensures that the patient's medical records are intact, despite the nonreturn of released radiographs to the lending facility.

THE DARKROOM

How film is handled in the darkroom can have a profound effect on the radiographs produced in a department. Common hazards to radiographic quality that can be found in the darkroom are white-light exposure, safelight exposure, ionizing radiation exposure, and other potential hazards.

Darkrooms must be free from all outside white-light exposure. A white-light source may be located inside the darkroom, but it should be connected to an interlock system whereby the film bin may not be opened as long as the darkroom white-light source is on.

Safelights used in the darkroom must be equipped with a safelight filter that is appropriate for the type of film(s) being handled in the darkroom. Commonly used filters include Kodak Wratten 6B for blue-sensitive film and Kodak GBX for ortho-chromatic film, which is sensitive to both blue-violet and green visible light. Safelight filters must be free of cracks because white light that leaks from the safelight could expose the film. The power rating of the light bulbs used in safelights should be no greater than that which is recommended by film manufacturers (generally 7.5 to 15 W) and that which is indicated on the outside of the box of radiographic film.

Ionizing radiation exposure to film in the darkroom is a potential hazard because many darkrooms share common walls with radiographic rooms. The walls that are common with the darkroom and a radiographic room must be lined with lead as required by law for standard protection from radiographic exposures. The film bin where film is stored and available for immediate use should also be lined with lead to prevent fog that may result from radiation exposure.

Other potential hazards to film in the darkroom include heat and chemical exposure. Film stored within the darkroom should not be near any heat source. Processing chemicals must be kept away from film and film-handling areas to prevent exposure and contamination of these areas.

The darkroom should be centrally located to radiographic rooms so they can be accessed quickly. Although the radiologists' reading area may be some distance away, there should be some film-viewing capability near the darkroom to allow radiographers to assess their radiographs immediately after processing.

Darkrooms may be equipped with a single door, a revolving door, or a maze access. The color of interior walls should be light to reflect the small amount of light available from safelights. Floors should be of some material that makes them nonslippery when wet if chemicals or water spill or leak inside the darkroom.

Unfortunately, darkrooms are not given much space within most radiology departments, so work space and storage space must be maximized. Countertops for film handling while cassettes are loaded and unloaded must be free of clutter.

Countertops must be clean and static free to avoid the formation of radiographic artifacts on the films. There are several brands of commercial cleaning fluid that contain an antistatic component ideal for cleaning darkroom countertops and processor feed trays. In addition, the floor space of the darkroom must be free of stored objects that one could trip over in the darkened environment.

Darkroom and Processor Quality Control

A quality control program must be implemented and systematically followed to ensure proper processing of radiographic film. A good quality control program should include steps for monitoring all of the equipment and activities required for the production of quality radiographic images. Radiographic quality cannot be achieved when film is improperly stored, mishandled before or after exposure, or incorrectly processed (See Table 8-4).

TABLE 8-4   QUALITY CONTROL FOR THE DARKROOM AND AUTOMATIC PROCESSOR

Quality Control Test	Schedule	Standards
Darkroom environment	Daily	Maintained clean, well ventilated, organized and safe
Safelight Test	Semiannually	Less than + 0.05 optical density added as fog
Automatic Processor Temperature	Weekly	Should not vary more than $\pm\, 0.5^\circ\, F$ $(0.3\,^\circ C)$
Replenishment Rates	Weekly	Should fall within $\pm\, 5\%$ of manufacturer's specification for replenishment type
Developer Solution pH	Quarterly	Maintained between $10 - 11.5$
Fixer Solution pH	Quarterly	Maintained between $4 - 4.5$
Developer Specific Gravity	Quarterly	Should not vary by more than $\pm\, 0.004$ from manufacturer's specifications
Processor Control Chart Monitoring	Daily	Speed and contrast indicators should not vary more than $\pm\, 0.15$ optical density from baseline measurements

Silver Recovery

Because fixer solution is used to remove unexposed silver halide from the film, used fixer solution contains a high concentration of accumulated silver. Silver is considered a heavy metal, and disposing of it is regulated by local and state agencies. In many locales, strict limits are placed on the concentrations of silver in used fixer that can be disposed into the sewer system. Some type of silver recovery must be done when radiographic processing accumulates high concentrations of silver. **Silver recovery** refers to the removal of silver from used fixer solution. For some facilities that regularly process large volumes of radiographs, the financial rewards of silver recovery may be an added incentive.

The most basic and simple method of silver recovery is to drain used fixer into a holding tank or container for retrieval by a silver recycler. This method is most appropriate for facilities that process a low volume of radiographs. The recycler must make regular visits to the facility or be called to retrieve the used fixer when the holding tank or container is full.

Silver-recovery units are available for on-site silver recovery and generally require servicing by an outside contractor who is familiar with the equipment and its method of removing silver. These silver-recovery units are connected directly to the drain system of the fixer tank to remove silver as used fixer solution passes through the unit. After the silver has been recovered, the used fixer is drained.

Silver-recovery units work by one of two methods. One method of silver recovery is called *metallic replacement*. Metallic replacement silver-recovery units can be one of two types: one that uses steel wool and one that uses a silver-extraction filter. A steel wool metallic replacement unit uses steel wool to filter the used fixer solution. Silver replaces the iron in the steel wool and can then be removed easily after significant accumulation in a canister or replacement cartridge occurs. A silver-extraction–type unit uses a foam filter that is impregnated with steel wool. Again, the silver from used fixer solution replaces the iron in the steel wool. A silver-extraction filter is more efficient at removing silver from used fixer and lasts longer than a simple steel wool metallic replacement unit.

Another method of silver recovery is the electrolytic method. It is the most efficient method, but the units needed for this process are also more expensive than metallic replacement units. Electrolytic units have an electrically charged drum or disk that attracts silver. The silver plates onto the drum or disk and can be removed when a substantial amount of silver has been collected.

Radiographic Artifacts

An **artifact** is any unwanted image on a radiograph. Artifacts are detrimental to radiographs because they can make visibility of anatomy, a pathologic condition, or patient identification information difficult or impossible. They decrease the overall radiographic quality of the image. Artifacts can be classified as *plus density* and *minus density*. Plus-density artifacts are greater in density than the area of the radiograph immediately surrounding them. Plus-density artifacts that are not caused by processing problems are presented in Table 8-5. Minus-density artifacts are of less density than the area of the radiograph immediately surrounding them. Some minus-density artifacts not caused by processing problems are presented in Table 8-6. For artifacts that result from processing problems, refer to Table 8-3.

TABLE 8-5   **SOME COMMON PLUS-DENSITY ARTIFACTS NOT CAUSED BY PROCESSING**

Artifact	Cause
Half-moon marks (Figure 8-16)	Bending or kinking of film
Scratches, abrasions (Figure 8-17)	Fingernail or other scratches
Static discharges (Figure 8-18)	Sliding films over flat surface
Fogging	Exposure to white light, ionizing radiation, heat, safelight fogging; expired film
Density outside of collimated area	Off-focus or "off-stem" radiation

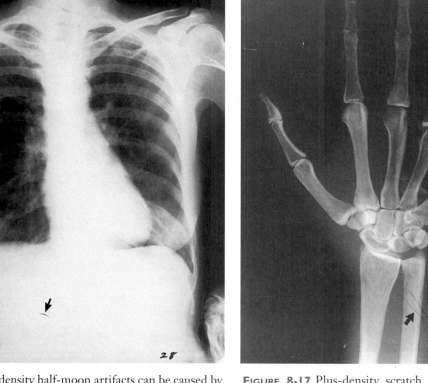

FIGURE 8-16 Plus-density half-moon artifacts can be caused by bending or kinking the film *(arrows)*.

FIGURE 8-17 Plus-density scratch artifacts can be caused by a fingernail *(arrow)*.

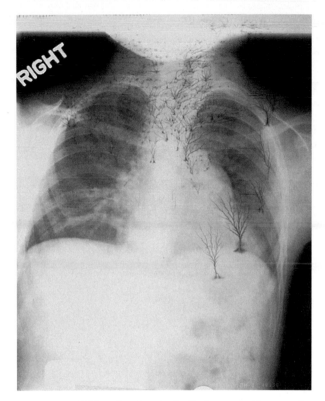

FIGURE 8-18 Plus-density static discharge artifact can be caused by sliding a film over a flat surface.

TABLE 8-6	SOME COMMON MINUS-DENSITY ARTIFACTS
Artifact	**Cause**
Fingerprints (Figure 8-19)	Moisture on finger transferred to film before exposure
Scratches, abrasions (Figure 8-20)	Scraping or removing emulsion
Foreign object (Figure 8-21)	Some unintended object in the imaging chain
Nonspecific density decrease (Figure 8-22)	Dirty screens or cassette

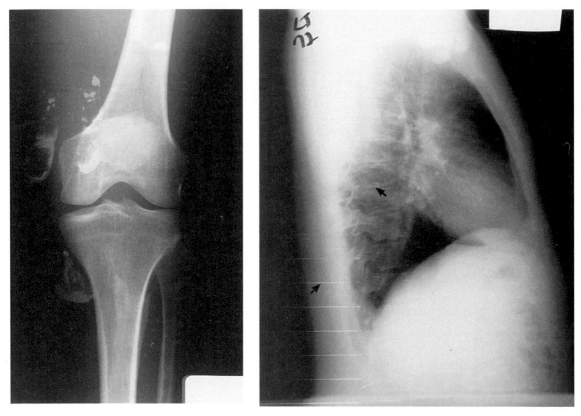

FIGURE 8-19 Minus-density caused by moisture on finger.

FIGURE 8-20 Minus-density scratch artifacts can be caused by transport rollers *(arrows)*.

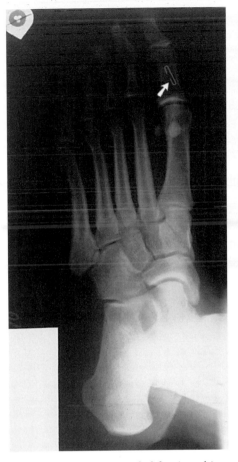

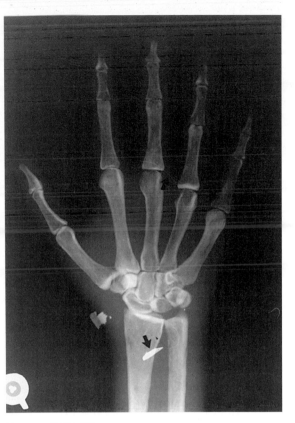

FIGURE 8-22 Dirty screens or cassettes can cause nonspecific minus density artifacts *(arrow)*.

FIGURE 8-21 An unintended foreign object on the radiograph results in a minus-density artifact

Review Questions

1. Conversion of the latent image to the manifest image is accomplished by
   A. the Gurney-Mott theory.
   B. radiographic processing.
   C. diffusion.
   D. oxidation.

2. The sequential order for processing radiographic film is
   A. developing, washing, fixing, drying.
   B. fixing, washing, developing, drying.
   C. developing, fixing, washing, drying.
   D. fixing, developing, washing, drying.

3. Which of the following solutions are responsible for reducing the exposed silver halide crystals to black metallic silver: (1) ammonium thiosulfate, (2) hydroquinone, or (3) phenidone?
   A. 1 and 2 only
   B. 1 and 3 only
   C. 2 and 3 only
   D. 1, 2, and 3

4. The chemical responsible for maintaining the alkalinity of the developing solution is
   A. sodium carbonate.
   B. phenidone.
   C. acetic acid.
   D. sodium sulfite.

5. The fixing agent used to clear the undeveloped silver halide crystals is
   A. hydroquinone.
   B. aluminum chloride.
   C. potassium bromide.
   D. ammonium thiosulfate.

6. Staining or fading of the permanent image results when too much _____ remains on the film with improper washing.
   A. phenidone
   B. acetic acid
   C. thiosulfate
   D. glutaraldehyde

7. Finished radiographs should retain what percentage of their moisture?
   A. 2% to 5%
   B. 10% to 15%
   C. 20% to 30%
   D. 35% to 45%

8. The type of roller responsible for moving the film from the bottom of the tank upward is a(n) _____ roller.
   A. transport
   B. entrance
   C. turnaround
   D. crossover

9. The type of roller responsible for moving the film from one tank to another is a(n) _____ roller.
   A. transport
   B. entrance
   C. turnaround
   D. crossover

10. Processing chemicals must be replenished to maintain activity and volume when depleted primarily by
    A. oxidation.
    B. diffusion.
    C. precipitation.
    D. condensation.

11. Decreasing the developer temperature
    A. decreases oxidation.
    B. increases contrast.
    C. decreases density.
    D. increases processing time.

12. Under what environmental conditions should radiographic film be stored?
    A. Temperature between 40° and 60° F and relative humidity between 40% and 60%
    B. Temperature between 50° and 70° F and relative humidity between 50% and 70%
    C. Temperature between 40° and 60° F and relative humidity between 50% and 70%
    D. Temperature between 50° and 70° F and relative humidity between 40% and 60%

13. Safelight filters are chosen based on the
    A. amount of light intensity.
    B. dimensions of the darkroom.
    C. film sensitivity.
    D. power rating.

14. The type of silver-recovery unit that uses an electrically charged drum to attract the silver is called a(n) _____ unit.
    A. an extraction filter
    B. electrolytic
    C. steel wool
    D. metallic replacement

15. A common plus-density artifact caused from bending the film is.
    A. half-moon marks.
    B. static discharge.
    C. abrasion.
    D. fogging.

CHAPTER 9

Sensitometry

1 Define all of the key terms in this chapter.

2 State all of the important relationships in this chapter.

3 Explain the importance of sensitometry to radiography.

4 Define *optical density* and explain its logarithmic scale.

5 State the diagnostic range of optical densities.

6 Given an optical density, convert it to its percentage of light transmission.

7 Explain the construction of sensitometric curves.

8 Identify all regions of a sensitometric curve.

9 Describe the characteristics of sensitometric curves.

10 Differentiate among the film characteristics of speed, contrast, and latitude.

11 Given sensitometric curves, compare their characteristics.

12 Calculate film speed and average gradient.

13 Evaluate the effect of exposure technique on the film characteristics of density and contrast.

KEY TERMS

sensitometry
intensity of radiation exposure
penetrometer
step-wedge densities
sensitometer
sensitometer strip
densitometer
optical density (OD)
logarithmic scale
base plus fog (B + F)
sensitometric curve
log relative exposure
toe region
D_{min}
straight-line region

shoulder region
D_{max}
speed
speed point
speed exposure point
antilog
film contrast
slope
gradient point
average gradient
gamma
exposure latitude
optimal density
maximum contrast
dynamic range

In radiography, **sensitometry** is the study of the relationship between the intensity of radiation exposure to the film and the amount of blackness produced after processing (density). The **intensity of radiation exposure** is the measurement of the quantity of radiation reaching an area of the film.

Use of Sensitometry

Sensitometry provides a method of evaluating the characteristics of film and film-screen combinations used in radiography. Radiographic film and intensifying screen manufacturers are capable of designing film and screens to respond differently to a given intensity of radiation exposure. Film and screens designed for radiography of the chest or extremities respond differently to equal amounts of radiation exposure. The radiographer should understand how the film and film-screen system that is used will respond to a given intensity of exposure.

Sensitometry is also a method of evaluating the performance of automatic processors. Because automatic processors affect a radiograph's density and contrast, the variability of their performance can be monitored by sensitometric methods.

Equipment

Several pieces of equipment are needed to evaluate the relationship between the intensity of radiation exposure and the density produced after processing. The radiographic film should be exposed to a range of radiation intensities to evaluate its response to low, middle, and high exposures. This can be accomplished easily by using a radiographic x-ray unit and passing the radiation through an object that varies in thickness. The resultant effect is an image of varying uniform densities that correspond to a specific intensity of radiation exposure.

PENETROMETER

A **penetrometer** is a device constructed of uniform absorbers of increasing thicknesses, such as aluminum or tissue-equivalent plastic (Figure 9-1). When radiographed, the penetrometer produces a series of uniform densities that resemble a step wedge (Figure 9-2). When **step-wedge densities** are produced with a penetrometer and a radiographic x-ray unit, the variability of the output of the equipment could affect the range of densities produced.

SENSITOMETER

A device known as a **sensitometer** is designed to produce consistent step-wedge densities by eliminating the variability of the x-ray unit (Figure 9-3). It uses a

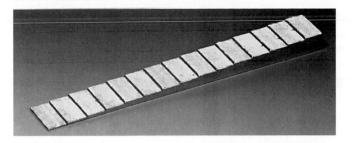

FIGURE 9-1 Penetrometer. When radiographed, a penetrometer produces an image showing a series of uniform densities.

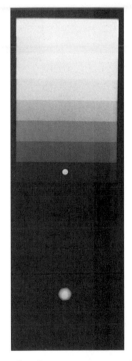

FIGURE 9-2 Radiograph of a penetrometer showing step-wedge densities.

controlled light source to expose an optical step-wedge template. The step-wedge template transmits light in varying intensities to expose the radiographic film. After the film has been processed, a density step-wedge image, or **sensitometric strip**, is produced. Penetrometers and sensitometers are available in 11-, 15-, or 21-step densities.

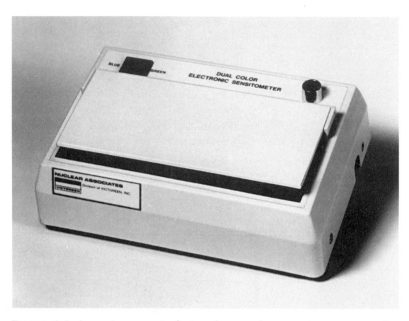

FIGURE 9-3 A sensitometer is designed to produce consistent step-wedge densities.

DENSITOMETER

A **densitometer** is a device used to numerically determine the amount of blackness on the film after processing (i.e., it measures radiographic density). This device is constructed to emit a constant intensity of light (incident) onto an area of film and then measure the amount of light transmitted through the film (Figure 9-4). The densitometer determines the amount of light transmitted and calculates a measurement known as **optical density (OD).**

Optical Density

Optical density is a numeric calculation that compares the amount of light transmitted through an area of radiographic film to the amount of light originally striking (incident) the film. Box 9-1 shows the mathematical formula used.

Box 9-1 *Light Transmittance Formula*

$$\frac{I_t}{I_o} \times 100$$

where I_t represents the amount of light transmitted and I_o represents the amount of original light incident on the film.

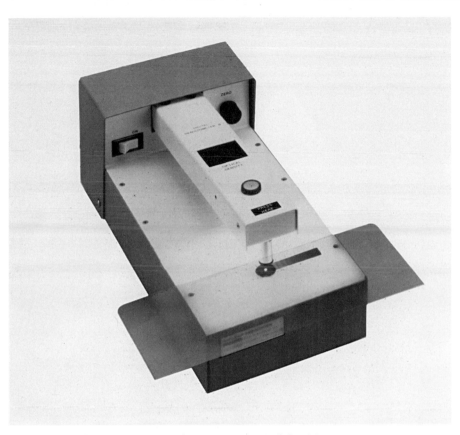

Figure 9-4 A densitometer is used to measure optical densities.

Because the range of radiographic densities is large, the calculation of radiographic densities is compressed into a **logarithmic scale** (Table 9-1) for easier management.

A film that allows 100% of the original incident light to be transmitted has a logarithmic value of 0. A film that allows only 1% of the original incident light through has a logarithmic value of 2.0. This logarithmic value of light transmittance is termed *optical density*. The formula used to calculate optical density is shown in Box 9-2.

TABLE 9-1   PERCENTAGE OF LIGHT TRANSMITTANCE AND CALCULATED OPTICAL DENSITIES

Percentage of Light Transmitted ($I_t/I_o \times 100$)	Fraction of Light Transmitted (I_t/I_o)	Optical Density (log I_o/I_t)
100	1	0
50	$1/2$	0.3
32	$8/25$	0.5
25	$1/4$	0.6
12.5	$1/8$	0.9
10	$1/10$	1
5	$1/20$	1.3
3.2	$4/125$	1.5
2.5	$1/30$	1.6
1.25	$1/80$	1.9
1	$1/100$	2
0.5	$1/200$	2.3
0.32	$2/625$	2.5
0.125	$1/800$	2.9
0.1	$1/1000$	3
0.05	$1/2000$	3.3
0.032	$1/3125$	3.5
0.01	$1/10,000$	4

Box 9-2 *Optical Density Formula*

$$\text{Optical density} = \text{Log}_{10} \frac{I_o}{I_t}$$

where I_o represents the amount of original light incident on the film and I_t represents the amount of transmitted light.

Important Relationship

Light Transmittance and Optical Density

As the percentage of light transmitted decreases, the optical density increases; as the percentage of light transmitted increases, the optical density decreases.

Notice the relationship between light transmittance and optical density. When 100% of the light is transmitted, the optical density equals 0.0. When 50% of the light is transmitted, the optical density is equal to 0.3, and when 25% of the light is transmitted, the optical density equals 0.6. When a logarithmic scale base 10 is used, every 0.3 change in optical density corresponds to a change in the percentage of light transmitted by a factor of 2 ($\log_{10}$ of 2 = 0.3).

Important Relationship

Optical Density and Light Transmittance

For every 0.3 change in optical density, the percentage of light transmitted has changed by a factor of 2. A 0.3 increase in optical density results from a decrease in the percentage of light transmitted by half, whereas a 0.3 decrease in optical density results from an increase in the percentage of light transmitted by a factor of 2.

Optical densities can range from 0.0 to 4.0 OD. Because most radiographic film has a tint added to its base and processing adds a slight amount of fog, the lowest amount of optical density is usually between 0.10 and 0.20 OD. This minimum amount of density on the radiographic film is termed the **base plus fog (B + F).**

DIAGNOSTIC RANGE

The useful range of optical densities is between 0.25 and 2.5 OD. However, the diagnostic range of optical densities for general radiography usually falls between 0.5 and 2.0 OD. This desired range of optical densities is found between the extreme low and high densities produced on the film.

Sensitometric Curve

When the optical density measurements from a sensitometric strip are graphed on semilogarithmic paper, the result is a curve characteristic of the radiographic film type. Box 9-3 lists other terms used for the **sensitometric curve.**

Box 9-3 *Other Terms for Sensitometric Curve*

Characteristic curve
D log E curve
H & D curve
Hurter & Driffield curve

    This sensitometric curve visually demonstrates the relationship between the intensity of radiation exposure (x axis) and the resultant optical densities (y axis) (Figure 9-5). The position of the curve on the x axis and its shape can vary greatly and depends on the type of radiographic film used.

LOG OF RELATIVE EXPOSURE

When sensitometric methods are used to evaluate the characteristics of radiographic film, it is more useful to measure the intensity of radiation exposure in increments of a constant change, such as doubling or halving. For every doubling or halving change in the percentage of light transmitted, a 0.3 change in optical density occurs. Along the x axis, for every 0.3 change in **log relative exposure,** the intensity of radiation exposure changes by a factor of 2 (Figure 9-6). When Figure 9-6 is used as an example, the relative mAs (the product of milliamperage and exposure time) value is 32 for the log exposure of 1.5, and the relative mAs value is 64 for the log of exposure 1.8. This relationship can be demonstrated throughout the log relative exposure scale on the sensitometric curve. Two exposures, one double the other, will always be separated by 0.3 on the logarithmic exposure scale.

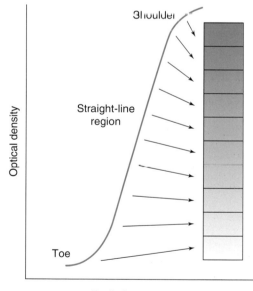

FIGURE 9-5 Plotting optical densities corresponding to the change in intensity of exposure results in a curve characteristic of the type of the film.

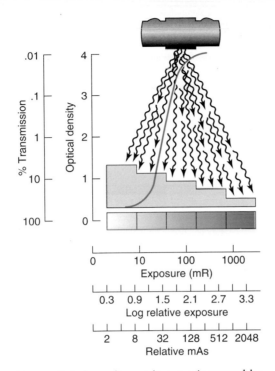

FIGURE 9-6 A sensitometric curve is created by plotting the optical density values obtained from the range of exposures that are used to create the step-wedge densities. The log relative exposure value representing the change in exposure by a factor of 2 is a more useful value than the milliroentgen (mR) exposure or relative mAs.

Important Relationship

Log Relative Exposure

A 0.3 change in log of exposure represents a change in intensity of radiation exposure by a factor of 2. An increase of 0.3 log of exposure results in a doubling of the amount of radiation exposure, whereas a decrease in 0.3 log of exposure results in halving the amount of radiation exposure.

REGIONS

A sensitometric curve demonstrates three distinct regions (Figure 9-7). When the characteristics of different types of radiographic film are evaluated, differences will be demonstrated within any of these regions.

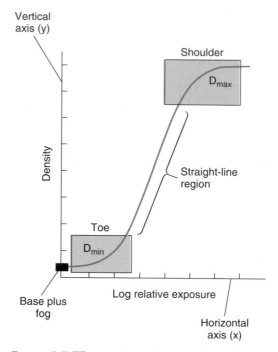

FIGURE 9-7 The sensitometric curve demonstrates three distinct regions: toe, straight-line, and shoulder.

Toe Region

The **toe region** of the sensitometric curve represents the area of low density. The point on the sensitometric curve where the minimum amount of radiation exposure produced a minimum amount of optical density is known as D_{min}. Generally, the D_{min} will be equal to B + F even though they represent two different measurements. Changes in exposure intensity in this region have little effect on the optical density.

Straight-Line Region

At some point along the x axis, changes in exposure begin to have a much greater effect on the optical density. This **straight-line region** is where the diagnostic or most useful range of densities is produced.

Shoulder Region

There is a point on the sensitometric curve where changes in exposure intensity no longer affect the optical density. In this **shoulder region,** the point on the curve where maximum density has been produced is known as D_{max}. Once the maximum density achievable within the film has been reached (D_{max}), continued increases in exposure intensity begin to reverse the amount of optical density. This process is called *solarization*, and it is the process used in the design of duplicating film.

Film Characteristics

Comparing sensitometric curves on these regions provides information about three important characteristics of the radiographic film. Each film characteristic plays an important role in radiographic imaging.

SPEED

An important characteristic of radiographic film is its sensitivity to radiation exposure, which is referred to as its **speed.** The speed of a film indicates the amount of optical density produced for a given amount of radiation exposure. It is a characteristic of the film's sensitivity to the intensity of radiation exposure.

Important Relationship

Film Speed and Optical Density

For a given exposure, as the speed of a film increases, the optical density produced also increases; as the speed of a film decreases, the optical density decreases.

Speed Point

The speed of radiographic film typically is determined by locating the point on a sensitometric curve that corresponds to the optical density of 1.0 plus B + F. This point is called the **speed point** (Figure 9-8). This optical density point is used because it is within the straight-line portion of the sensitometric curve. The speed point serves as a standard method of indicating film speed.

Speed Exposure Point

When comparing film types, the radiographer must determine what log of exposure produced the speed point. This can be determined by drawing a line from the sensitometric curve speed point to the area on the x axis (log of exposure) that produced the optical density at 1.0 plus B + F (Figure 9-9). This important point, called the **speed exposure point**, indicates the intensity of exposure needed to produce a density of 1.0 plus B + F (speed point). A film that has a speed exposure point of 0.9 is faster than a film having a speed exposure point of 1.2.

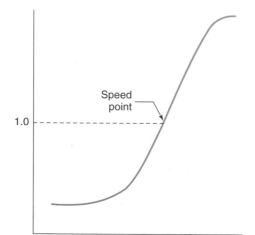

FIGURE 9-8 The sensitometric curve speed point indicates the intensity of exposure needed to produce a density of 1.0 plus base plus fog.

FIGURE 9-9 The speed exposure point indicates the intensity of exposure needed to produce a density of 1.0 plus base plus fog (speed point).

Important Relationship

Film Speed and Speed Exposure Point

The lower the speed exposure point, the faster the film speed; the higher the speed exposure point, the slower the film speed.

Figure 9-10 presents two sensitometric curves and their respective speed point and speed exposure point. A faster-speed film is positioned to the left (closer to the y axis) of slower-speed film.

Practical Tip

Sensitometric Curves Position along the X Axis

Sensitometric curves of faster-speed film are positioned to the left of slower-speed film, and sensitometric curves of slower-speed film are positioned to the right of faster-speed film.

It is important to remember that the speed of the film is determined by the amount of exposure (log of exposure) needed to produce an optical density of 1.0 plus B + F, regardless of the shape of the sensitometric curve (Figure 9-11).

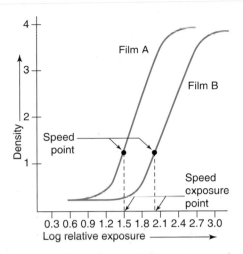

FIGURE 9-10 Obtaining the same speed point requires that *Film A* have a 1.5 log of exposure and *Film B* have a 2.0 log of exposure. Faster-speed films are located to the left of slower-speed films.

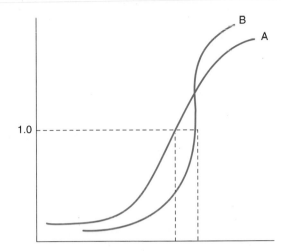

FIGURE 9-11 As the shape of the sensitometric curve varies, the speed can also vary if it is measured at points other than the standard of 1.0 plus base plus fog.

Film Speed Formula

The radiographer needs to comprehend the method used to compare various film speeds and their subsequent effect on exposure techniques. The film speed formula provides a mathematical calculation for the differences in film speed (Box 9-4).

Comparison of speed among different types of film will assist the radiographer in determining the changes needed in exposure technique to maintain comparable radiographic density. Calculating the **antilog** of the differences between two speed exposure points demonstrates the factorial change in intensity of exposure.

For example, the antilog of the exposure difference between Film A and Film B equals 2.24 (see Box 9-4). This represents a change in log of exposure by a factor of 2.24, or 224%. This means that Film B is 2.24 times faster than Film A. To maintain density when changing from Film B to Film A, the radiographer must increase the exposure technique by a factor of 2.24 (Film B mAs [20] × 2.24 = 44.8 new mAs for Film A).

This formula also can be used to calculate changes in exposure to alter the optical density for a given radiographic image: calculate the difference between the exposure points for the initial optical density point and the desired optical density point and find the antilog. As in the previous example with two different types of film, the antilog can be used to adjust the actual mAs to increase or decrease the optical densities on a repeated radiographic study.

> **Box 9-4** *Film Speed Formula*
>
> $$\text{Antilog } (E_2 - E_1)$$
>
> | **Film A** | **Film B** |
> |---|---|
> | $E_2 = 1.2$ | $E_1 = 0.85$ |
>
> $$\text{Antilog } (1.2 - 0.85)$$
>
> Antilog $(0.35) = 2.24$. Film B is 2.24 times faster than Film A. This factorial change in intensity can then be applied to the actual mAs value to adjust the optical density accordingly.

X Mathematical Application

Using Sensitometry to Calculate Exposure Technique Changes

60 mAs produced an image density of 2.05 (log E = 1.54). What mAs would produce an image density of 1.30 (log E = 1.38)?

Subtract log E of the original density (2.05) from the log E of the desired density (1.30):

$$
\begin{array}{r}
1.38 \\
-1.54 \\
\hline
-0.16; \text{ antilog of } -0.16 = \ 0.69
\end{array}
$$

Multiply the original mAs by 0.69:

$$60 \text{ mAs} \times 0.69 = 41.4 \text{ mAs}$$

Changing the original optical density on the repeat radiograph from 2.05 to 1.30 requires the mAs to be decreased to 41.4.

CONTRAST

Radiographic contrast is a result of both the subject contrast and the **film contrast.** Film contrast is controlled by the design and manufacturing of the film components and the effect of processing. The ability of a radiographic film to provide a level of contrast can be evaluated by the steepness, or **slope,** of the sensitometric curve. The slope of this line mathematically indicates the ratio of the change in *y* (optical density) for a unit change in *x* (log relative exposure) (Box 9-5).

Visually comparing the steepness (slope) of the straight-line region of the curve provides a method of evaluating the level of contrast produced by a film (Figure 9-12). Radiographic film capable of producing higher contrast will have a more vertical straight-line region (steeper slope).

Important Relationship

Slope and Film Contrast

The steeper the slope of the straight-line region (more vertical), the higher the film contrast; the lesser the slope (less vertical), the lower the film contrast.

Box 9-5 *Determining the Slope of a Line*

$$\text{Slope} = \frac{Y \text{ (rise)}}{X \text{ (run)}} , \frac{y_2 - y_1}{x_2 - x_1}$$

The slope of a line mathematically indicates its tilt or slant. Comparisons of the slope (mathematical calculation) can be made among different lines. For radiography, the higher the number, the steeper the slope, and the lower the number, the lesser the slope.

General-purpose radiographic film is categorized as either high contrast or medium contrast.

Gradient Point

Determining the slope along any portion of the sensitometric curve provides information about the contrast produced at that point, which is called the **gradient point.** Gradient points can be determined for any region of the sensitometric curve, such as the toe, middle, and shoulder. The gradient point can be determined by calculating the slope of the line (change in optical density divided by the change in log exposure) at any portion of the curve.

Average Gradient

When comparing film, the radiographer typically determines contrast by calculating the sensitometric curve's **average gradient** of the slope of the straight-line region (Figure 9-13). A standard used in sensitometry is to determine the film contrast between the optical densities of 0.25 and 2.0 plus B + F. Finding the difference between these two points and dividing by the difference between their respective log of exposures provides a numerical calculation for film contrast. Most radiographic film has an average gradient between 2.5 and 3.5.

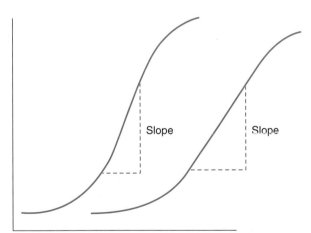

FIGURE 9-12 The slope of the straight-line region determines the inherent film contrast. Steeper slopes indicate higher contrast.

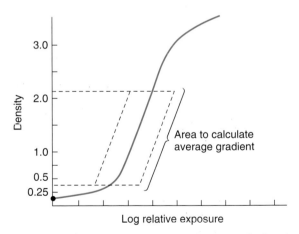

FIGURE 9-13 A film's average gradient is calculated between a low density (0.25 plus base plus fog) and a high density (2.0 plus base plus fog).

Mathematical Application

Calculating Average Gradient

$$\text{Average gradient} = \frac{D_2 - D_1}{E_2 - E_1}$$

where

$D_1 = \text{OD } 0.25 + 0.17 \text{ (B + F)}$
$D_2 = \text{OD } 2.0 + 0.17 \text{ (B + F)}$
$E_1 = \text{Exposure that produces } D_1$
$E_2 = \text{Exposure that produces } D_2$

Example:

$$\frac{2.17 - 0.42}{1.46 - 0.8} = \frac{1.75}{0.66} = 2.65 \text{ Average gradient}$$

Film contrast is higher for a film with an average gradient of 3.0 compared with that of a film having an average gradient of 2.7.

Important Relationship

Average Gradient and Film Contrast

The greater the average gradient, the higher the film contrast; the lower the average gradient, the lower the film contrast.

Gamma

Gamma is another gradient point that is calculated from points surrounding the optical density of 1.0 found within the straight-line region of the sensitometric curve.

Gradient point, average gradient, and gamma all provide information about the contrast produced by a type of radiographic film. To make equal comparisons of the characteristics of film, the radiographer must determine the contrast by using the same method.

EXPOSURE LATITUDE

Exposure latitude refers to the range of exposures that produce optical densities within the straight-line region of the sensitometric curve (Figure 9-14). Radiographic films that are capable of responding to a wide range of exposures to produce optical

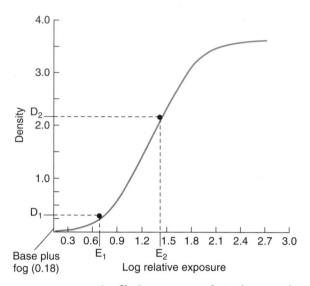

FIGURE 9-14 A film's exposure latitude can be determined by finding the range of exposures that will produce densities within the straight-line region of the curve. Using a low and high density similar to those used to calculate average gradient would provide optical densities within the straight-line region of the sensitometric curve.

densities within the straight-line region are considered wide-latitude film. When comparing a film with narrow latitude to one with wide latitude, it is apparent that a film with narrow latitude is a higher-contrast film and a film with wide latitude is a lower-contrast film (Figure 9-15). A steep slope has a small range of exposures available to produce densities within the straight-line region, whereas a less steep slope has a greater range of densities available to produce densities within the straight-line region.

Important Relationship

Exposure Latitude and Film Contrast

Exposure latitude and film contrast have an inverse relationship. High-contrast radiographic film has narrow latitude, and low-contrast film has wide latitude.

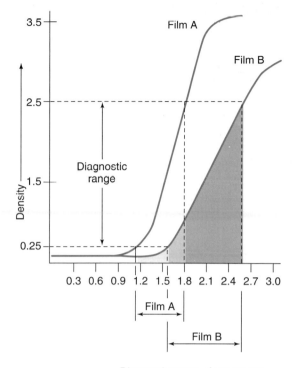

FIGURE 9-15 A higher-contrast film, *Film A*, has a narrower range of exposures available to produce optical densities within the straight-line region compared with a lower-contrast film, *Film B*.

When selecting a type of radiographic film to use, the radiographer should evaluate its characteristics in terms of speed, contrast, and latitude. Radiographic film used in chest radiography typically requires lower contrast and wider-exposure latitude, whereas film designed for use with skull radiography requires higher contrast, resulting in narrow-exposure latitude. The speed of radiographic film is considered in combination with the intensifying screen speed to provide a film-screen system speed.

Clinical Considerations

To provide radiographic images of optimal radiographic quality, the radiographer must control visibility factors of density and contrast appropriately. A relationship exists between density and contrast to maximize the amount of recorded detail visible.

OPTIMAL DENSITY

For a given anatomic area to be radiographed, exposure techniques selected should produce radiographic densities that lie within the straight-line region of the sensitometric curve. Optical densities within this range maximize the amount of information visible within the radiographic image, resulting in **optimal density.**

The challenge for radiographers is to determine the amount of radiation exposure necessary to produce optical densities within the straight-line region of a film's sensitometric curve. Different types of radiographic film may require different amounts of exposure to produce optical densities within the straight-line region. As demonstrated previously, it may take more or less radiation exposure to produce an optical density of 1.0 plus B + F for Film A as compared with Film B. Therefore the relationship between radiation exposure and optical density depends on the shape and position of a film's sensitometric curve.

For a given type of radiographic film, when optical densities lie within the straight-line region of the sensitometric curve, a change in exposure technique has a direct effect on optical density (Figure 9-16). When optical densities lie outside the range of the straight-line region, a greater or lesser change in exposure technique may be needed to move the optical densities back within the diagnostic range (0.5 to 2.0 OD). When evaluating a radiograph with a density error, the radiographer must determine the amount of change needed in the exposure to place the optical densities within the diagnostic range.

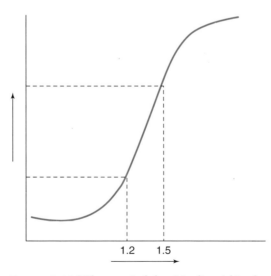

FIGURE 9-16 When optical densities lie within the straight-line region of the curve, a 0.3 change in log exposure (change by a factor of 2) produces a direct effect in optical densities.

Changes in Exposure Technique to Correct for Density Errors

To correct for the density error, optical densities that lie outside the straight-line region of the sensitometric curve (toe or shoulder region) require a greater or lesser change in exposure than those that lie within the straight-line region.

In diagnostic radiology one type of film is typically used for most procedures. Access to a film's sensitometric curve for the purpose of calculating exposure changes is not practical. Therefore it is the radiographer's responsibility to use the standard guidelines (discussed in Chapter 4) regarding exposure changes to correct for density errors.

MAXIMUM FILM CONTRAST

Film contrast is the difference in optical density between two points anywhere along the sensitometric curve (Figure 9-17). If these differences in optical density were plotted as points between the x and y axes, the result would be a film's contrast curve (Figure 9-18). When the contrast curve is evaluated, it is apparent that **maximum contrast** (the greatest difference in optical densities) is achievable within the straight-line region of the sensitometric curve. When optical densities of the anatomic area of interest lie outside the straight-line region, film contrast is decreased.

Achieving Maximum Film Contrast

To achieve the maximum contrast that the film is capable of producing, the radiographer must ensure that the optical densities lie within the straight-line region of the sensitometric curve.

When optical densities lie within the straight-line region of the sensitometric curve, the film has reached its maximum capability in visualizing recorded detail.

In summary, sufficient radiographic density is needed to visualize recorded detail. A film's maximum radiographic contrast can be visualized only when optical densities lie within the straight-line region of the sensitometric curve. When optical densities lie outside the straight-line region, film contrast is decreased. When both optimum density and maximum contrast have been achieved, the visibility of recorded details is of optimal radiographic quality.

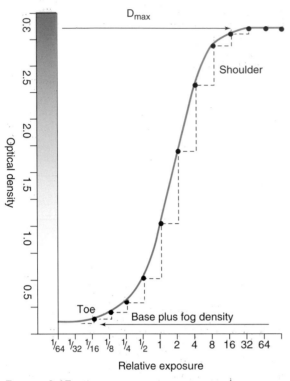

FIGURE 9-17 Density differences calculated along the sensitometric curve can be used to evaluate film contrast.

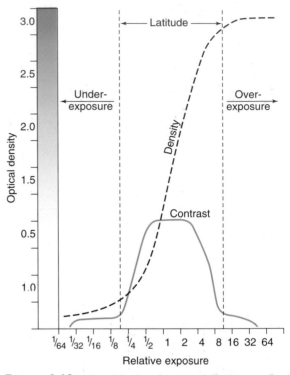

FIGURE 9-18 Plotting the density differences of a sensitometric curve results in a contrast curve. Maximum film contrast is achieved within the straight-line region.

Digital Imaging

The response of a digital image receptor to the intensity of radiation exposure is different when compared with that of radiographic film. The digital image receptor is more responsive to the wide range of x-ray intensities exiting the anatomic part. In addition, a digital imaging system can retain significantly more information than radiographic film. The information received from the digital image receptor and processed in the computer represents the **dynamic range** capabilities of the digital system. Dynamic range refers to the shades of gray (range of densities) that can be displayed within the digital image. The greater the number of shades of gray available to create an image, the wider the dynamic range of the imaging system. Digital imaging systems have the ability to visually display a wider range of densities than film radiography. Figure 9-19 compares film and digital image receptors and their response to the range of x-ray intensities.

As evidenced by the sensitometric curve for film, x-ray intensities must fall within a smaller range to display radiographic densities that can be visible. The linear response of a digital image receptor results in a greater range of densities available for display within the digital image. The digital image can display a shade of gray that represents low x-ray intensity, as well as medium and high x-ray intensities.

In addition, the digital imaging system can manipulate the density differences to change the scale of contrast. The ability of the digital image receptor to respond to a wider range of x-ray intensities and visually display a greater range of densities is a significant advantage of digital imaging.

Like film-screen radiography, exposure factors used in digital imaging are selected to produce an optimal quality image. However, the wide dynamic range capability of digital imaging systems allows for some exposure error adjustment. Refer to Chapter 12 for a more detailed discussion of digital imaging.

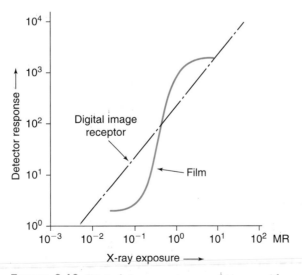

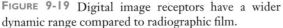

FIGURE 9-19 Digital image receptors have a wider dynamic range compared to radiographic film.

Review Questions

1. What term is defined as a measurement of the amount of light transmitted through the film?
   A. Sensitometry
   B. Film contrast
   C. Film speed
   D. Optical density

2. What is the diagnostic range of optical densities?
   A. 0.15 to 4.0
   B. 0.5 to 1.25
   C. 0.50 to 2.0
   D. 0.10 to 2.0

3. An optical density of 1.0 indicates that _____ light was transmitted.
   A. 0.01%
   B. 0.1%
   C. 1.0%
   D. 10%

4. A _____ change in optical density results from a change in the percentage of light transmittance by a factor of 2.
   A. 0.03
   B. 0.3
   C. 3.0
   D. 30

5. Changes in exposure have little effect on density in which of the following regions of the sensitometric curve: (1) toe, (2) shoulder, or (3) straight line?
   A. 1 and 2 only
   B. 1 and 3 only
   C. 2 and 3 only
   D. 1, 2, and 3

6. When the exposure technique used produces densities outside the straight-line portion of a sensitometric curve, how is contrast affected?
   A. Increased
   B. No effect
   C. Decreased
   D. Improved

7. Compare the sensitometric curves in
   Figure 9-20. Which film is faster?
   A. Film A
   B. Film B
   C. Film C
   D. Film D

8. Compare the sensitometric curves in
   Figure 9-20. Which film has lower contrast?
   A. Film A
   B. Film B
   C. Film C
   D. Film D

9. Film B has an exposure speed point of 1.5, and
   Film A has an exposure speed point of 1.2. Is
   there a difference in speed?
   A. Film A is twice as fast as Film B.
   B. Film A and B have equal speed.
   C. Film A is half as fast as Film B.
   D. Film B is twice as fast as Film A.

10. Changes in radiation exposure have the greatest
   effect on optical densities in which
   sensitometric region?
   A. Toe
   B. Shoulder
   C. Straight-line
   D. Toe and Shoulder

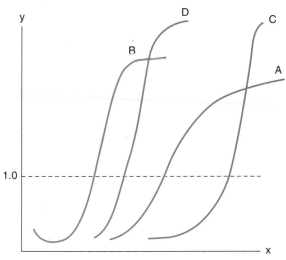

FIGURE 9-20

Exposure Factor Selection

1 Define all of the key terms in this chapter.

2 State all of the important relationships in this chapter.

3 State the purpose of exposure technique charts and the conditions surrounding their use.

4 Describe the characteristics of technique charts.

5 Differentiate between variable kVp/fixed mAs and fixed kVp/variable mAs technique charts.

6 Identify advantages and disadvantages of variable kVp and fixed kVp charts.

7 Recognize the steps involved in developing an exposure technique chart.

exposure technique charts
calipers
variable kVp/fixed mAs technique chart
fixed kVp/variable mAs technique chart

optimal kVp
extrapolated
comparative anatomy

The radiographer has the primary task of selecting the exposure factors that produce a quality radiographic image. Many variables can affect the production of a quality radiograph. Previous chapters have discussed the exposure factors and their effect on the radiographic image. Knowledge of these factors and of the qualities inherent in an optimal radiographic image aids the radiographer in the selection of exposure factors for a particular radiographic examination. Exposure technique charts are useful tools that assist the radiographer in selecting a manual exposure technique or when using automatic exposure control (AEC). Exposure technique charts are equally valuable for film-screen or digital image receptors. This chapter focuses on the design and use of exposure technique charts to assist the radiographer in the consistent production of quality radiographic images.

Exposure Technique Charts

Exposure technique charts are preestablished guidelines used by the radiographer to select standardized manual or AEC exposure factors for each type of radiographic examination. Technique charts standardize the selection of exposure factors for the typical patient so that the quality of radiographic images is consistent.

For each radiographic procedure, the radiographer consults the technique chart for the recommended exposure variables—kilovoltage peak (kVp), mAs (the product of milliamperage and exposure time), type of image receptor, grid, and source-to-image receptor distance (SID). Based on the thickness of the anatomic part to be radiographed, the radiographer selects the exposure factors presented in the technique chart. For example, if a patient is scheduled for a routine abdominal examination, the radiographer positions the patient and aligns the central ray (CR) to the patient and image receptor, measures the abdomen for a manual technique, and consults the chart for the predetermined standardized exposure variables.

Because many factors have an impact on the selection of appropriate exposure factors, technique charts are instrumental in the production of consistent quality radiographs, reduction in repeat radiographic studies, and reduction in patient exposure. The proper development and use of technique charts are keys to the selection of appropriate exposure factors.

Important Relationship

Exposure Technique Charts and Radiographic Quality

A properly designed and used technique chart standardizes the selection of exposure factors to help the radiographer produce consistent quality radiographs while minimizing patient exposure.

CONDITIONS

A technique chart presents exposure factors that are to be used for a particular examination based on the type of radiographic equipment. Technique charts help ensure that consistent image quality is achieved throughout the entire radiology department; they also decrease the number of repeat radiographic studies needed and therefore decrease the patient's exposure.

Technique charts do not replace the critical thinking skills required of the radiographer. The radiographer must continue to use individual judgment and discretion in properly selecting exposure factors for each patient and type of examination. The radiographer's primary task is to produce the highest quality radiograph while delivering the least amount of radiation exposure. Technique charts are designed for the average or typical patient and do not account for unusual circumstances. These atypical conditions require accurate patient assessment and appropriate exposure technique adjustment by the radiographer.

Practical Tip

Technique Chart Limitations

Exposure technique charts are designed for the typical or average patient. Patient variability in terms of body build or physical condition, or the presence of a pathologic condition, requires the radiographer to problem solve when selecting exposure factors.

A technique chart should be established for each x-ray tube, even if a single generator is used for more than one tube. For example, if a radiographic room has two x-ray tubes, one for a radiographic table and one for an upright Bucky unit, each tube should have its own technique chart because of possible inherent differences in the exposure output produced by each tube. Each portable radiographic unit must also have its own technique chart.

For technique charts to be effective tools in producing consistent quality radiographs, departmental standards for radiographic quality should be determined. In addition, standardization of exposure factors and the use of accessory devices are needed. For example, the adult knee can be radiographed adequately with or without the use of a grid. Although both radiographs might be acceptable, departmental standards may specify that the knee be radiographed with the use of a grid. These types of decisions should be made before technique chart development takes place so that the departmental standards can be clarified. Technique charts are then constructed using these standards, and radiographers should adhere to the departmental standards.

Two conditions must be met for technique charts to be effective. First, the radiographic equipment for which the charts are developed must be calibrated. Calibration ensures that the kVp, milliamperage (mA), and exposure time settings are accurate. Second, image processing must be consistent throughout the department to produce the proper radiographic density and contrast. Poor radiographic quality could result from inconsistencies in processing or from the radiographic equipment being out of calibration, rather than the improper selection of exposure factors. A good quality control program for all radiographic equipment will ensure monitoring of any variability in the equipment's performance.

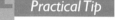

Practical Tip

Equipment Performance

Radiographic equipment must be operating within normal limits for technique charts to be effective.

Accurate measurement of part thickness is a critical condition for the effective use of technique charts. The measured part thickness determines the selected kVp and mAs values for the radiographic examination. If the part is measured inaccurately, incorrect exposure factors may be selected. Measurement of part thickness must be standardized throughout the radiology department.

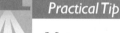

Practical Tip

Measurement of Part Thickness

Accurate measurement of part thickness is critical to the effective use of exposure technique charts.

Calipers are devices that measure part thickness and should be readily accessible in every radiographic room (Figure 10-1). In addition, the technique chart should specify the exact location for measuring part thickness. Part measurement may be performed at the location of the CR midpoint or the thickest portion of the area to be radiographed. Errors in part thickness measurement are one of the more common mistakes made when one is consulting technique charts.

DESIGN CHARACTERISTICS

Technique charts can vary widely in terms of their design, but they share some common characteristics. The primary exposure factors of kVp and mA, and common accessory devices used, such as image receptor type and grid ratio, are included regardless of the type of technique chart used. The exposure factors that should be standardized in technique charts are listed in Box 10-1.

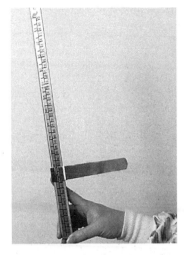

FIGURE 10-1 A caliper is used to measure part thickness.

From Mosby's radiographic instructional series: radiographic imaging, St Louis, 1998, Mosby.

Box 10-1 *Contents Standardized in a Technique Chart*

Anatomic part	Grid ratio
Automatic exposure control detector selections, if applicable	Kilovoltage peak
	Milliamperage
Central ray location	Part thickness and measuring point
Type of image receptor	Position or projection
Focal spot size	Source-to-image receptor distance

Types of Technique Charts

Two primary types of exposure technique charts exist: fixed kVp/variable mAs and variable kVp/fixed mAs. Each type of chart has different characteristics, and both have advantages and disadvantages. Technique charts can be differentiated by the need for measurement precision, contrast scale and its variability, patient dose, and heat load on the x-ray tube (Table 10-1).

TABLE 10-1 **EXPOSURE TECHNIQUE CHART CHARACTERISTICS**

Design Type	Part Measurement	Contrast Scale	Radiographic Contrast	Patient Dose	Tube Heat Load
Variable kVp/ fixed mAs	Critical	Shorter	Variable	Higher	Increased
Fixed kVp/ variable mAs	Less critical	Longer	Standardized	Lower	Decreased

---

VARIABLE KVP/FIXED MAS TECHNIQUE CHART

The **variable kVp/fixed mAs technique chart** is based on the concept that kVp can be increased as the anatomic part size increases. Specifically, the baseline kVp is increased by 2 for every 1-cm increase in part thickness, whereas the mAs is maintained (Table 10-2). The baseline kVp is the original kVp value predetermined for the anatomic area to be radiographed. The baseline kVp is then adjusted for changes in part thickness.

Accurate measurement of part thickness is critical to the effective use of this type of technique chart. Part thickness must be measured accurately to ensure that the 2-kVp adjustment is applied appropriately. The radiographer consults the technique chart and prepares the exposure factors specified for the type of radiographic examination (i.e., mAs, SID, grid use, and type of image receptor). The anatomic part is measured accurately and the kVp is adjusted appropriately. For example, a standard exposure technique for a patient's knee measuring 10 cm is 63 kVp at 20 mAs, 400 speed image receptor, and use of a 12:1 table Bucky grid. A patient with a knee measuring 14 cm would then require a change only in the kVp, from 63 to 71 (2 kVp change for every 1-cm change in part thickness).

> *Important Relationship*
>
> *Variable kVp/Fixed mAs Technique Chart*

The variable kVp chart adjusts the kVp for changes in part thickness while maintaining a fixed mAs.

TABLE 10-2 VARIABLE KILOVOLTAGE/FIXED mAs TECHNIQUE CHART

Anatomic part	**Knee**	Image receptor	**400 speed**
Projection	**AP**	Table top/Bucky	**Bucky**
Measuring point	**Midpatella**	Grid ratio	**12:1**
Source-to-image receptor distance	**40 inches**	Focal spot size	**Small**

cm	kVp	mAs
10	63	20
11	65	20
12	67	20
13	69	20
14	71	20
15	73	20
16	75	20
17	77	20
18	78	20

Determination of the baseline kilovoltage for each anatomic area has not been standardized. Historically, a variety of methods have been used to determine the baseline kVp value. The goal is to determine a kVp value that adequately penetrates the anatomic part when using a 2-kVp adjustment for every 1-cm change in tissue thickness. The baseline kVp value can be determined experimentally with the use of radiographic phantoms (patient equivalent devices).

Developing a variable kVp technique chart that can be used effectively throughout the kilovoltage range has proved problematic. In addition, technology advances in imaging receptors may challenge the applicability of the variable kVp/fixed mAs type technique chart.

In general, changing the kVp values for variations in part thickness may be ineffective throughout the entire range of radiographic examinations. A variable kVp/fixed mAs chart may be most effective when small extremities, such as hands, toes, and feet, are being imaged. At low kVp levels, small changes in kVp may be more effective than changing the mAs.

Practical Tip

Applicability of a Variable kVp/Fixed mAs Technique Chart

Variable kVp technique charts may be more effective when small extremities are being imaged.

This type of chart has the advantage of being easy to formulate because making exposure changes to compensate for different part sizes is simple. However, because kVp is variable, radiographic contrast may vary as well, and these types of charts tend to be less accurate for part size extremes. Adequate penetration of the part is not necessarily assured, and radiographs produced with the use of this type of chart tend to have higher radiographic contrast.

FIXED kVp/VARIABLE mAs TECHNIQUE CHART

The **fixed kVp/variable mAs technique chart** (Table 10-3) uses the concept of selecting an optimal kVp value that is required for the radiographic examination and adjusting the mAs for variations in part thickness. **Optimal kVp** can be described as the kVp value that is high enough to ensure penetration of the part but not too high to diminish radiographic contrast. For this type of chart, the optimal kVp value for each part is indicated, and mAs is varied as a function of part thickness.

> ### Important Relationship
>
> *Fixed kVp/Variable mAs Technique Charts*
>
> Fixed kVp/variable mAs technique charts identify optimal kVp values and alter the mAs for variations in part thickness.

TABLE 10-3 **FIXED KILOVOLTAGE/VARIABLE mAs TECHNIQUE CHART**

Anatomic part	**Knee**	Image receptor	**400 speed**
Projection	**AP**	Table top/Bucky	**Bucky**
Measuring point	**Midpatella**	Grid ratio	**12:1**
Source-to-image receptor distance	**40 inches**	Focal spot size	**Small**

cm	kVp	mAs
10-13	73	10
14-17	73	20
18-21	73	40

Optimal kVp values required for each anatomic area have not been standardized. Although charts identifying common kVp values for different anatomic areas can be found, experienced radiographers tend to develop their own optimum kVp values. The goal is to determine the kVp that will penetrate the part without compromising radiographic contrast. Specifying the optimal kVp value used in a fixed kVp/variable mAs technique chart encourages all radiographers to adhere to the departmental standards.

Once optimal kVp values are established, fixed kVp/variable mAs technique charts alter the mAs for variations in thickness of the anatomic part. A general guideline is for every 4- to 5-cm change in part thickness, the mAs should be adjusted by a factor of 2. Using the previous example for a patient's knee measuring 10 cm and an optimal kVp, the exposure technique would be 73 kVp at 10 mAs, 400 speed image receptor with a 12:1 table Bucky grid. A patient with a knee measuring 14 cm would then require a change only in the mAs, from 10 to 20 (a 4-cm increase in part thickness requires a doubling of the mAs).

Accurate measurement of the anatomic part is important but is less critical compared with the precision needed with variable kVp charts. An advantage of fixed kVp/variable mAs technique charts is that patient groups can be formed around 4- to 5-cm changes. Patient thickness groups can be created instead of listing thickness changes in increments of 1 cm.

Practical Tip

Fixed kVp/Variable mAs and Part Measurement

Accuracy of measurement is less critical with fixed kVp/variable mAs technique charts than with variable kVp/fixed mAs technique charts.

The fixed kVp/variable mAs technique chart has the advantages of easier use, more consistency in the production of quality radiographs, greater assurance of adequate penetration of all anatomic parts, standardization of radiographic contrast, and increased accuracy with extreme variation in size of the anatomic part.

Exposure Technique Chart Development

Radiographers can develop effective technique charts that will assist in exposure technique selection. The steps involved in technique chart development are similar, regardless of the design of the technique chart. The primary tools needed are radiographic phantoms, calipers for accurate measurement, and a calculator. Once optimal radiographs are produced using these phantoms, exposure techniques can be **extrapolated** (mathematically estimated) for imaging other similar anatomic areas.

A critical component in technique chart development is to determine minimum kVp value that will adequately penetrate the anatomic part to be radiographed. One method available is to use the concept of **comparative anatomy**, which can assist the radiographer in determining minimum kVp values. This concept states that different parts of the same size can be radiographed by use of the same exposure factors, provided that the minimum kVp value needed to penetrate the part is used in each case. For example, a radiographer knows what exposure factors to use with a particular radiographic unit for a knee that measures 10 cm in the anteroposterior (AP) aspect, but he or she is now confronted with radiographing a shoulder. The radiographer measures the shoulder in the AP aspect and determines that it measures 10 cm. The radiographer does not have a technique for a shoulder for this radiographic unit. The concept of comparative anatomy states that the shoulder in this case can be radiographed successfully using the same technique that the radiographer has used for the 10-cm knee as long as the minimum kVp to penetrate the part has been used for the shoulder or knee.

DEVELOPMENT STAGES

The stages for development of exposure technique charts are similar regardless of the type of chart. Patient-equivalent phantoms for sample anatomic areas provide a means for establishing standardized exposure factors. Using the concept of comparative anatomy assists the radiographer in extrapolating exposure techniques for similar anatomic areas. After the initial development of an exposure technique chart, the chart must be tested for accuracy and revised if necessary.

The first task is to determine the type of technique chart that will be used in the department. The type of technique chart selected determines the baseline kVp level. Typically, variable kVp/fixed mAs technique charts use a lower kVp value than fixed kVp/variable mAs technique charts.

During initial technique chart development, several phantom radiographs are produced to demonstrate a range of quality radiographs. All of the radiographs must be reviewed, and the radiographs deemed unacceptable according to departmental standards should be eliminated. The goal is to determine the baseline exposure techniques to be used to produce quality radiographs.

For variable kVp/fixed mAs technique charts, the remaining acceptable images should provide an upper and lower limit of kilovoltages to be used for the anatomic area. The kVp values for variations in part thickness by 1 cm must be determined by use of the extrapolation technique.

For fixed kVp/variable mAs technique charts, the acceptable radiograph using the highest kVp value should be selected, or selected based on departmental standards. This radiograph represents the optimal kVp used for the anatomic area. The mAs values for variations in part thicknesses of 4 to 5 cm must be determined by use of the extrapolation technique. Box 10-2 provides an example.

Box 10-3 lists the development stages for an exposure technique chart.

An exposure technique chart must be tested and revised after its initial development. Poor radiographic quality may result when the exposure technique chart is not used properly. Radiographers need to problem solve by evaluating the numerous exposure variables that could have contributed to a poor-quality radiograph before assuming the chart is ineffective.

A commitment by management and staff to use exposure technique charts is critical to the consistent production of quality radiographs. Well-developed technique charts are of little use if radiographers choose not to consult them.

Box 10-2 *Example of How to Develop a Fixed kVp/Variable mAs Exposure Technique Chart*

Step 1 Pelvis phantom is positioned on the radiographic table for an anteroposterior (AP) projection of the right hip. The central ray (CR) is at the midpoint of the hip, the source-to-image receptor distance (SID) is 40 inches, and collimation is to film size. The part was measured (26 cm) at the CR entrance point. Select initial exposure technique factors based on departmental standards.

Step 2 Using the kVp/mAs 15% rule, the following five radiographs are produced:
1. 51 kVp at 200 mAs
2. 60 kVp at 100 mAs
3. 70 kVp at 50 mAs
4. 81 kVp at 25 mAs
5. 93 kVp at 12.5 mAs

Step 3 Radiographs 1 and 5 are deemed unacceptable.

Step 4 Radiograph 3 is selected as optimum based on departmental standards.

Step 5 The following technique chart is developed by extrapolating the exposure techniques (variable mAs) for changes in part thickness.

Anatomic part	**Hip**	Image receptor	**400 speed**
Projection	**AP**	Table top/Bucky	**Bucky**
Measuring point	**CR entrance**	Grid ratio	**12:1**
SID	**40 inches**	Focal spot size	**Small**

cm	kVp	mAs
16-19	70	12.5
20-23	70	25
24-27	70	50
28-31	70	100
32-35	70	200

> **Box 10-3**   *How to Develop an Exposure Technique Chart*
>
> 1. Select a kVp value appropriate to the anatomic area to be radiographed. Determine the mAs value that produces the desired radiographic density.
> 2. Using a patient-equivalent phantom, produce several radiographs, varying the kVp and mAs values. Use the general rules for exposure technique adjustment (i.e., the 15% rule). Radiographic densities should be similar.
> 3. Evaluate the quality of the radiographs, and eliminate those deemed unacceptable.
> 4. Of the remaining acceptable radiographs, select those having the kVp value appropriate for the type of technique chart desired and according to departmental standards.
> 5. Extrapolate the exposure techniques (variable kVp or variable mAs) for changes in part thickness.
> 6. Use the concept of comparative anatomy to develop technique charts for similar anatomic areas.
> 7. Test the technique chart for accuracy, and revise if needed.

Review Questions

1. What is defined as preestablished guidelines used to select standardized exposure factors?
   - **A.** Comparative anatomy
   - **B.** Extrapolation technique
   - **C.** Exposure technique chart
   - **D.** Automatic exposure control

2. _____ is the primary patient factor that determines the selection of exposure factors.
   - **A.** Age
   - **B.** Part measurement
   - **C.** Physical condition
   - **D.** Weight

3. A primary goal of exposure technique charts is to
   - **A.** extend the life of the x-ray tube.
   - **B.** improve the radiographer's accuracy.
   - **C.** consistently produce quality images.
   - **D.** increase the patient work flow.

4. Which of the following is an important condition required for technique charts to be effective?
   - **A.** Equipment must be calibrated to perform properly.
   - **B.** One technique chart should be used for all radiographic units.
   - **C.** All technologists should use the same mA setting.
   - **D.** The chart should not be revised once it has been used.

5. Which of the following factors would *not* be standardized on technique charts?
   - **A.** Image receptor speed
   - **B.** Grid ratio
   - **C.** SID
   - **D.** Patient age

6. What type of exposure technique system uses a fixed mAs regardless of part thickness?
   - **A.** Fixed kVp
   - **B.** Variable kVp
   - **C.** Manual
   - **D.** AEC

7. Of the following, which is most important when using a technique chart?
   - **A.** One radiographer revises the chart.
   - **B.** A high mA value is set.
   - **C.** The part is measured accurately.
   - **D.** Patient history is included.

8. What is an advantage of the fixed kVp technique chart?
   - **A.** It produces higher-contrast images.
   - **B.** It reduces patient exposure.
   - **C.** kVp changes are easy to make.
   - **D.** Smaller technique changes are possible.

9. What is a disadvantage of the variable kVp technique chart?
   - **A.** It produces lower-contrast images.
   - **B.** It is difficult to construct.
   - **C.** It may not be effective with small extremities.
   - **D.** It increases heat load on the x-ray tube.

10. In creating either type of exposure technique chart, what is most important?
   - **A.** Achieving adequate penetration of the anatomic part
   - **B.** Selecting the same milliamperage value
   - **C.** Not requiring radiographers to consult them
   - **D.** Producing images with similar radiographic contrast

CHAPTER 11

Automatic Exposure Control

Automatic exposure control (AEC) is one method for setting exposure factors to ensure that a quality radiographic image is produced. When setting a manual (not automatic) technique, the radiographer selects the kilovoltage peak (kVp), milliamperage (mA), and exposure time based on many factors, including source-to-image receptor distance (SID), the thickness and tissue type of the part, the pathology, and the image receptor. A technique chart helps standardize manual techniques. If the radiographer accurately assesses all variables involved in producing the radiograph and the technique chart is accurate, the resulting image should be of optimal quality. However, if the radiographer does not account for or misjudges a variable (forgetting to check the SID or not realizing that the patient has a pleural effusion), the resulting image will be suboptimal.

AEC systems are designed to produce radiographs (film-screen imaging) with optimal density by controlling the amount of radiation exposure reaching the film. When used correctly, AEC should produce consistently optimal density radiographs because, based on sensitometry, a specific amount of radiation to the film produces a specific density. If the x-ray exposure is terminated when the exposure corresponding to optimal density is reached, the resultant radiograph should demonstrate optimal density (Figure 11-1).

Important Relationship

X-Ray Exposure and Density

The amount of density on a film depends on the amount of radiation exposure reaching the film. The greater the exposure to the film, the greater the resulting density.

AEC systems must measure the radiation exposure reaching the image receptor; once a preset amount that corresponds to optimal density is reached, the systems shut off the x-ray timer, thereby terminating the radiation. Such a system makes it easier to produce consistent levels of radiographic density. AEC systems have limitations, however. The radiographer must be aware of several technical considerations to use AEC systems successfully. Another type of system, anatomic programming, sometimes is present on the same radiographic units as AEC systems and can assist in the selection of proper exposure factors.

Purpose

The relationship between AEC and density is critical for film-screen imaging but does not hold true for digital radiography where the digital image density or brightness is manipulated by the computer. However, AEC is still important for digital radiography because the amount of radiation exposure reaching the digital

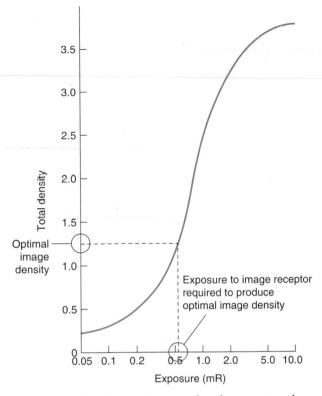

FIGURE 11-1 Sensitometric curve that demonstrates the relationship between x-ray exposure at the image receptor level and the resulting radiographic density. A specific amount of x-ray exposure must reach the image receptor to produce optimal image density.

image receptor is a key factor in digital image quality. The relationship between AEC and digital radiography is discussed at the end of the chapter.

AEC systems also are called *automatic exposure devices (AEDs)*, and sometimes they are erroneously referred to as *phototiming*. **Automatic exposure control (AEC)** is a system used to consistently control radiographic density by terminating the length of exposure based on the amount of radiation reaching the image receptor. There are many thousands of possible combinations of kVp, mA, SID, exposure time, film-screen system speeds, and grid ratios. When combined with patients of various sizes and with various pathologic conditions, the selection of proper exposure factors becomes a difficult task. Technique charts make setting technical factors much more manageable, but there are always patient factors that require the radiographer's assessment and judgment. When using AEC systems, the radiographer must still use individual discretion to select an appropriate kVp, mA, film-screen system, and grid. However, the AEC device will determine the exposure time (and therefore total exposure) that is used. AEC is not a panacea, but it can make obtaining optimal radiographic densities significantly less difficult.

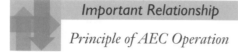

Important Relationship

Principle of AEC Operation

Once a predetermined amount of radiation is transmitted through a patient, the x-ray exposure is terminated. This determines the exposure time and therefore the resulting density.

AEC Systems

All AEC devices work by the same principle of operation: radiation is transmitted through the patient and converted into an electrical signal, terminating the radiographic exposure. This occurs when a predetermined amount of radiation has been detected, as indicated by the level of electrical signal that has been produced. The difference in AEC systems lies in the type of device that is used to convert radiation into electricity. Two types of AEC systems have been used: those that use photomultiplier tubes and those that use ionization chambers. Photomultiplier tube systems represent the first generation of AEC systems used in radiography, and it is from this type of system that the term *phototiming* has evolved. *Phototiming* specifically refers to the use of an AEC device that uses photomultiplier tubes, even though these systems are not common today. Therefore the use of the term *phototiming* is usually in error. The more common type of AEC system in use today uses ionization chambers. Regardless of the specific type of AEC system used, almost all systems use a set of three radiation-measuring detectors, arranged in some specific manner (Figure 11-2). The radiographer selects the configuration of these devices, determining which one(s) of the three actually measures radiation exposure reaching the image receptor. These devices are variously referred to as *sensors, chambers, cells, pick-ups,* or *detectors.* These radiation-measuring devices are referred to here for the remainder of the discussion as **detectors.**

Important Relationship

Radiation-Measuring Devices

Detectors are the AEC devices that measure the amount of radiation transmitted. The radiographer selects which of the three detectors to use.

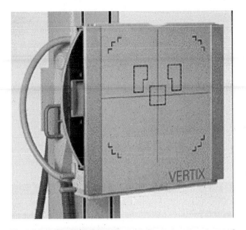

FIGURE 11-2 The size and arrangement of the three AEC detectors are clear on this upright chest stand.

PHOTOMULTIPLIER TUBE SYSTEMS

A **photomultiplier (PM) tube** is an electronic device that converts visible light energy into electrical energy. Photomultiplier tube AEC devices are considered exit-type devices because the detectors are positioned behind the cassette (Figure 11-3) so that radiation must exit the cassette before it is measured by the detectors. Light paddles serve as the detectors, and the radiation interacts with the paddles, producing visible light. This light is transmitted to remote PM tubes that convert this light into electricity. The timer is tripped and the radiographic exposure is terminated when a sufficiently large charge has been received. This electrical charge is in proportion to the radiation to which the light paddles have been exposed. PM tube systems have largely been replaced with ionization chamber systems.

IONIZATION CHAMBER SYSTEMS

An **ionization chamber,** or **ion chamber,** is a hollow cell that contains air and is connected to the timer circuit via an electrical wire. Ionization chamber AEC devices are considered entrance-type devices because the detectors are positioned in front of the cassette (Figure 11-4) so that radiation interacts with the detectors just before interacting with the cassette. When the ionization chamber is exposed to radiation from a radiographic exposure, the air inside the chamber becomes ionized, creating an electrical charge. This charge travels along the wire to the timer circuit. The timer is tripped and the radiographic exposure is terminated when a sufficiently large charge has been received. This electrical charge is in proportion to the radiation to which the ionization chamber has been exposed. Compared with PM tubes, ion chambers are less sophisticated and less accurate, but they are less prone to failure. Most of today's AEC systems use ionization chambers.

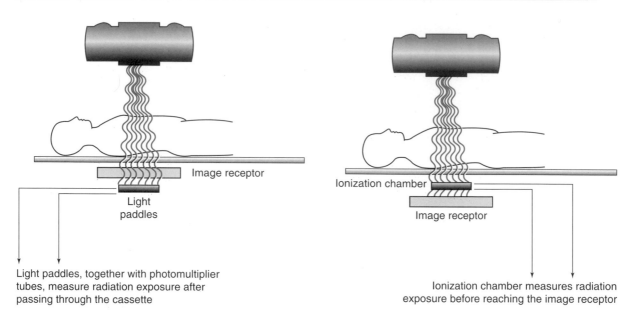

Light paddles, together with photomultiplier tubes, measure radiation exposure after passing through the cassette

Ionization chamber measures radiation exposure before reaching the image receptor

FIGURE 11-3 The photomultiplier tube AEC system has the light paddles (detectors) located directly below the image receptor. This is an exit-type device in that the x-rays must exit the image receptor before they are measured by the detectors.

FIGURE 11-4 The ionization chamber AEC system has the detectors located directly in front of the image receptor. This more modern system is termed *entrance-type* because the x-ray exposure is measured just before entering the image receptor.

Important Relationship

Function of the Ionization Chamber

The ionization chamber interacts with exit radiation before it reaches the image receptor. Air in the chamber is ionized, and an electric charge that is proportional to the amount of radiation is created.

Technical Considerations with AEC

To use AEC to its best advantage, radiographers must be aware of some important technical considerations peculiar to AEC systems.

CENTERING OF THE PART

Proper centering of the part being examined is crucial when using an AEC system. The anatomic area of interest must be centered properly over the detector(s) that the radiographer has selected. Improper centering of the part over the selected detector(s) produces a radiograph that is either underexposed or overexposed. For example, when an AEC device is used for a lateral lumbar spine image, if the central ray is too far posterior and the center detector is selected (as appropriate), the soft tissue will superimpose the detector rather than the spine. In this case the soft tissue behind the spine will demonstrate optimal density, but the spine itself will be underexposed (Figure 11-5). Inaccurate centering is probably the most common cause of suboptimal density when AEC is used.

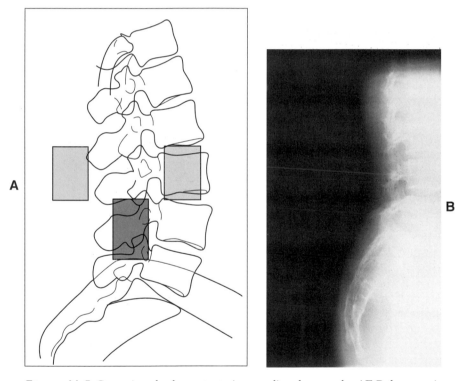

FIGURE 11-5 Centering the key anatomic area directly over the AEC detector is critical in producing optimal density radiographs. Whatever anatomic area is located over the detector has optimal density. **A,** With the center detector selected, the centering for this lateral lumbar spine is posterior to the lumbar vertebral bodies. The lamina, spinous processes, and soft tissue cover the detector. **B,** The resulting radiograph demonstrates appropriate density just posterior to the vertebral bodies, but the bodies themselves are underexposed. This radiograph is unacceptable because of inaccurate centering resulting in underexposure of the anatomy of interest.

DETECTOR SELECTION

Selection of the detector(s) to be used for a particular examination is critical when using an AEC system. The selected detectors actively measure radiation during exposure. Measuring radiation that passes through the anatomic area of interest is important. The general guideline is to select the detector(s) that will be superimposed by the anatomic structures that are of greatest interest and need to be visualized on the radiograph. Failure to use the proper detectors results in a radiograph that is either underexposed or overexposed. In the case of a posteroanterior (PA) chest radiograph, the area of radiographic interest includes the lungs and heart; therefore one or two outside detectors should be selected to place the detectors directly beneath the critical anatomic area. If the center detector were mistakenly selected, the anatomy superimposing this detector includes the thoracic spine. If the exposure is made, the resultant image will demonstrate optimal density in the spine, with the lungs overexposed (Figure 11-6). In the manual that accompanies the radiographic unit, manufacturers of AEC devices provide recommendations for which detectors to use for specific examinations. Recommendations for detector selection also can be found in many radiographic procedures textbooks.

Important Relationship

Accurate Part Centering and Detector Selection

Accurate centering and detector selection are critical with AEC systems because the radiograph will demonstrate optimal density of the anatomy located directly over the detector. If the area of radiographic interest is not directly over the selected detector, that area probably will be overexposed or underexposed.

KVP AND MA SELECTIONS

Because AEC controls only the radiographic density and has no effect on radiographic contrast, the kVp for a particular examination should be selected as it would be for that examination, regardless of whether an AEC device is used. The radiographer must select the kVp value that provides appropriate scale of contrast and is at least the minimum kVp to penetrate the part. In addition, the higher the kVp value used, the shorter the exposure time needed by the AEC device. Because high kVp radiation is more penetrating (reducing the total amount of x-ray exposure to the patient because more x-ray photons exit the patient) and the detectors are measuring quantity of radiation, the preset amount of radiation exposure is reached sooner with high kVp. The kVp selected should be high enough to produce the radiographic contrast appropriate to the part being examined while keeping the patient's exposure as low as possible.

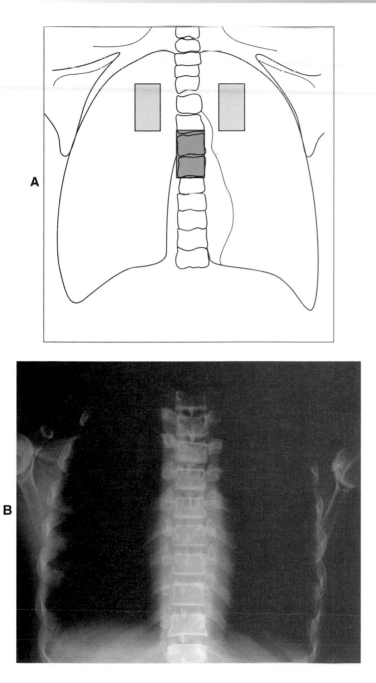

FIGURE 11-6 Selecting the detector(s) to be located directly under the critical anatomic area may make the difference between an optimal and unacceptable image. The posteroanterior (PA) chest should be imaged using both outside detectors to locate them directly under the lung tissue. **A,** This diagram shows that the center detector was inappropriately selected for the PA chest, placing the thoracic spine directly over the detector. **B,** The resulting chest radiograph demonstrates optimal density in the area of the spine, but the lungs are notably overexposed.

Practical Tip

AEC, kVp, and Radiographic Contrast

Assuming the radiographer is selecting or using a kVp value above the minimum needed to penetrate the part, adjustment of this value does not affect density when an AEC device is used. It does affect radiographic contrast, however (Figure 11-7). The radiographer must be sure to set the kVp value as needed to ensure adequate penetration and to produce the appropriate scale of contrast.

When the radiographer uses a control panel that allows the mA and time to be set independently, he or she should select the mA value as it would be for that particular examination, regardless of whether an AEC device is used. The mA value selected has a direct effect on the exposure time needed by the AEC device. Therefore, if the radiographer wants to decrease exposure time for a particular examination, he or she may easily do so by increasing the mA value. Increasing or decreasing the mA value does not affect the image density but does have a definite impact on the length of the exposure.

DENSITY SELECTIONS

AEC devices are equipped with density controls that allow the radiographer to fine-tune the radiographic density that is produced by the unit. These generally are in the

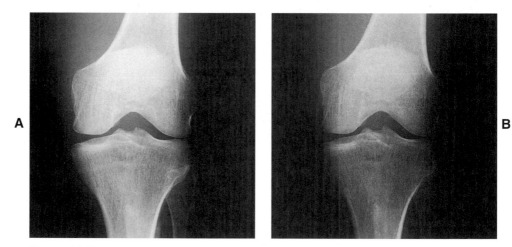

FIGURE 11-7 Adjustment of kVp with AEC examinations does not affect image density but does affect contrast. Both knees are imaged by use of the center detector, and all other factors are identical, except for the kVp value. **A,** Imaged at 55 kVp, this knee demonstrates a short scale of contrast. **B,** Imaged at 90 kVp, this image has a much longer scale of contrast, but the density remains essentially the same.

form of buttons on the control panel that are numbered −2, −1, +1, and +2. The actual numbers presented on density controls vary, but each of these buttons changes exposure time by some predetermined amount or increment expressed as a percentage. A common increment is 25%, meaning that the predetermined exposure level needed to terminate the timer can be either increased or decreased from normal in one increment (+25% or −25%) or two increments (+50% or −50%). Manufacturers usually provide information for their equipment on how these density controls should be used. Common sense and practical experience should also serve as guidelines for the radiographer.

Practical Tip

AEC and Density Settings

Routinely using plus or minus density settings to produce acceptable radiographs indicates that a problem exists, possibly a problem with the AEC device.

COLLIMATION

Collimation is a factor when AEC systems are used because the additional scatter radiation produced by failure to accurately restrict the beam may cause the detector to terminate the exposure prematurely. The detector is unable to distinguish transmitted radiation from scattered radiation and, as always, ends the exposure when a preset amount of exposure has been reached. Because the detector is measuring both types of radiation exiting the patient, the timer is turned off too soon when scatter is excessive, which results in underexposure of the area of interest. The radiographer should open the collimator to the extent that the part being radiographed is imaged appropriately, but not so much as to cause the AEC device to stop the exposure before the area being imaged is properly exposed.

BACKUP TIME

Backup time refers to the maximum length of time the x-ray exposure will continue when using an AEC system. The backup time may be set by the radiographer or controlled automatically by the radiographic unit. It may be set as backup exposure time or as backup mAs (the product of mA and exposure time). The role of the backup time is to act as a safety mechanism when an AEC system fails or the equipment is not used properly. In either case, the backup time protects the patient from receiving unnecessary exposure and protects the x-ray tube from reaching or exceeding its heat loading capacity.

Important Relationship

Function of Backup Time

Backup time, the maximum exposure time allowed during an AEC examination, serves as a safety mechanism when the AEC is not used or is not functioning properly.

The backup time might be reached as the result of operator oversight when an AEC examination, such as a chest x-ray, is done at the upright Bucky and the radiographer has set the control panel for table Bucky. The table detectors are forced to wait an excessively long time to measure enough radiation to terminate the exposure. In a case such as this, the backup time limits the patient's exposure and keeps the tube from overloading.

When controlled by the radiographer, the backup time should be set high enough to be greater than the exposure needed but low enough to protect the patient from excessive exposure in case of a problem. Setting the backup time at 150% to 200% of the expected exposure time is appropriate. If the backup timer periodically or routinely terminates the exposure, higher mA values should be used to shorten the exposure time.

Important Relationship

Setting Backup Time

Backup time should be set at 150% to 200% of the expected exposure time. This allows the properly used AEC system to appropriately terminate the exposure but protects the patient and tube from excessive exposure if a problem occurs.

THE PATIENT

Some patients may require greater technical consideration when AEC is used for their radiographic procedures. Abdominal examinations using AEC can be compromised if a patient has an excessive amount of bowel gas. If a detector is superimposed by an area of the abdomen with excessive gas, the timer will terminate the exposure prematurely, resulting in an underexposed radiograph. Likewise, destructive pathologic conditions can cause underexposure of the area of radiographic interest. The presence of positive contrast media, an additive pathologic condition, or a prosthetic device that superimposes the detector can cause excessive density.

The size, shape, and location of the anatomic area of interest also affect the use of AEC systems. If the area of radiographic interest does not completely cover the detector (e.g., the clavicle), the resulting density may be inappropriate. In addition, if the detector must be very close to the edge of the patient's body (e.g., shoulder or pediatric chest), the detector must be covered completely by the anatomic area of interest. If a portion of the detector is exposed directly by the x-ray beam, the radiation exposure level necessary to terminate the exposure is reached almost immediately, resulting in underexposure of the area of interest.

Important Relationship

The Patient and AEC

If the anatomic area directly over the detector does not represent the anatomic area of interest, inappropriate density may result. This can happen when the anatomic area over the detector contains a foreign object, a pocket of air, contrast media, or if the anatomic area does not completely cover the detector.

The radiographer must consider these circumstances individually and determine how best to image the patient or part. Using the density control buttons may work in some cases, whereas in others it may be necessary to recenter the patient or part. Sometimes the best solution is a manual technique determined through use of a technique chart. AEC is not a replacement for a knowledgeable radiographer using critical thinking skills.

BUCKY SELECTION

Many radiographic units have AEC devices in both the table Bucky and an upright Bucky. If more than one Bucky per radiographic unit uses AEC, the radiographer must be certain to select the correct Bucky before making an exposure. Failure to do so results in the patient and image receptor being exposed to excessive radiation. The backup time is reached, the exposure terminated, and a repeat radiographic study must be done, thereby increasing the patient's dose.

A similar problem can occur when not using a Bucky, such as with cross-table, tabletop, or stretcher/wheelchair studies. If the AEC system is activated with these types of examinations, an unusually long exposure results because the detectors are not being exposed to radiation. Again, the backup time will probably be reached and the patient's dose will be excessive. Some radiographic units are designed so that an exposure does not occur if the AEC device has been selected and there is no cassette detected in the Bucky.

Practical Tip

AEC and Non-Bucky Studies

The radiographer should be certain to deactivate the AEC system and use a manual technique when performing any radiographic study where the image receptor is located outside of the Bucky.

mAs Readout

When a radiographic study is performed using an AEC device, the total amount of radiation (mAs) required to produce the appropriate density is determined by the system. Many radiographic units include a mAs readout display, where the actual amount of mAs used for that image is displayed immediately after the exposure, sometimes for only a few seconds. It is critical for the radiographer to take note of this information when it is available. Knowledge of the mAs readout has a number of advantages. It allows the radiographer to become more familiar with manual technical factors. If the image is suboptimal, knowing the mAs readout provides a basis from which the radiographer can make exposure adjustments by switching to manual technique. There may be studies with different positions where AEC and manual technique are combined because of difficulty with accurate centering. For example, knowing the mAs readout for the anteroposterior (AP) lumbar spine gives the radiographer an option to switch to manual technique for the oblique exposures, making technique adjustments based on solid mAs information.

Practical Tip

AEC and mAs Readout

If the radiographic unit has a mAs readout display, the radiographer should be sure to notice the reading after the exposure is made. This information can be invaluable.

Limitations of AEC Systems

AEC systems are excellent at producing consistent levels of radiographic density when used properly, but the radiographer should also be aware of the technical limitations of using an AEC system.

Interchangeability of Film-Screen Systems

Different film-screen systems cannot be interchanged easily once an AEC device is calibrated to produce specific densities. When a radiographic unit with AEC is first installed, the AEC device is calibrated (and at intervals thereafter). The purpose of calibration is to ensure that consistent and appropriate radiographic densities are produced. When calibration is performed, it is done for a particular film-screen system speed. The AEC device cannot sense when the radiographer uses a different speed of film or screen and instead produces a density based on the system for which it was calibrated, resulting in either too much or too little density. For example, if a 100 speed film-screen system is used with an AEC device instead of the appropriate 400 speed film-screen system, the resulting image will have too little density because the exposure stopped (as preset) for the more sensitive 400 speed system. Some radiographic units have AEC devices that can accommodate more than one speed of film-screen system. With these types of units, the control panel indicates which film-screen system will be used for the next exposure.

MINIMUM RESPONSE TIME

The term **minimum response time** refers to the shortest exposure time that the system can produce. Minimum response time usually is longer with AEC systems than with other types of radiographic timers (i.e., other types of radiographic timers usually are able to produce shorter exposure times than AEC devices). This can be a problem with some segments of the patient population, such as pediatric patients and uncooperative patients. With pediatric patients and others who cannot or will not cooperate with the radiographer by holding still or holding their breath during the exposure, AEC devices may not be the technology of choice.

LACK OF CALIBRATION

For an AEC device to work properly, the radiographic unit and the AEC device must each be calibrated to accepted standards. Failure to maintain regular calibration of the unit and AEC device results in radiographs that lack consistent, reproducible, and appropriate density. This ultimately leads to overexposure of the patient and poor efficiency of the imaging department, as well as the possibility of improper interpretation of radiographs.

Anatomic Programming

Anatomic programming, or **anatomically programmed radiography (APR),** refers to a radiographic system that allows the radiographer to select a particular button on the control panel that represents an anatomic area; a preprogrammed set of exposure factors is displayed and selected for use. The appearance of these controls varies, depending on the unit (Figure 11-8), but the operation of all APR systems is based on the same principle. APR is controlled by an integrated circuit or computer chip that has been programmed with exposure factors for different projections and positions of different anatomic parts. Once an anatomic part and projection or position has been selected, the radiographer can adjust the exposure factors that are displayed.

APR and AEC are not related in their functions, other than as systems for making exposures. However, these two different systems are commonly combined on radiographic units because of their similar dependence on integrated computer circuitry. APR and AEC often are used in conjunction with one another. A radiographer can use APR to select a projection or position for a specific anatomic

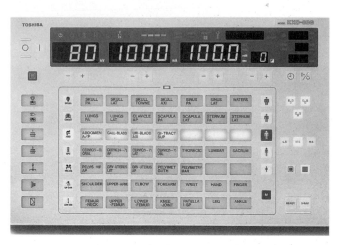

FIGURE 11-8 Anatomically programmed radiography selections are displayed on this console. The radiographer can choose from posteroanterior lungs, lateral skull, knee, and hand, among others. Each selection displays the preprogrammed technical factors that the radiographer can decide to use or adjust.

part and view the kVp, mA, and exposure time for an equivalent manual technique. The radiographer can then opt to use AEC to determine the exposure time. When APR is used in conjunction with AEC on some radiographic units, the APR system not only selects and displays manual exposure factors but also selects and displays the AEC detectors to be used for a specific radiographic examination. For example, pressing the Lungs PA button results in selection of 110 kVp, the upright Bucky, and the two outside AEC detectors. As with AEC, APR is a system that automates some of the work of radiography. However, the individual judgment and discretion of the radiographer is still required to use the APR system correctly for the production of optimal quality images.

AEC and Digital Radiography

Within a limited range, the amount of radiation exposure reaching a digital image receptor (IR) is manipulated by the computer to produce an image with appropriate brightness or density. However, the computer has definite limitations, and if AEC is not used appropriately, both image quality and the patient can suffer. If the digital IR is underexposed, the computer adjusts the density, but the image quality will be quite poor because of quantum mottle or noise. If the IR is overexposed, the computer attempts to adjust the density, but the decreased contrast and excessive patient exposure will have already occurred.

Because AEC controls the amount of radiation reaching the IR, appropriate use of AEC results in the digital IR receiving the correct amount of exposure and therefore enhances digital image quality. In addition, the patient is not overexposed to radiation in the process. Errors made in using AEC with digital radiography may result in appropriate density (because the computer makes adjustments), but image quality suffers because of overexposure or underexposure of the imaging plate (IP) and the patient may suffer because of overexposure to radiation.

Important Relationship

AEC and Digital Radiography

The radiographer must use AEC accurately when using digital imaging systems. Failure to do so can result in overexposure of the patient to ionizing radiation or production of an image that is of poor quality.

Practical Tip

AEC Calibration and Computed Radiography (CR)

As indicated in Chapter 7, the sensitivity of CR systems is approximately equivalent to a 200 speed film-screen system. In order to achieve optimal digital image quality, AEC devices used with CR image receptors should be recalibrated to ensure that the exposure to the IP is correct.

The following tables clarify the relationship between density and imaging variables for both film-screen (Table 11-1) and digital radiography (Table 11-2).

TABLE 11-1　FILM-SCREEN RADIOGRAPHY AND AEC

An upright PA chest exam done using the following factors produces an optimal image:

400 speed film-screen system	AEC with 2 outside detectors
110 kVp	upright Bucky
400 mA	0 (normal) density

Assuming all other factors remain the same, how would the following changes affect the density of the image?

Change	Effect on Density in Area of Interest	Explanation
100 speed IR	↓	The AEC is calibrated to the 400 speed system. The exposure ends when the exposure is sufficient for the 400 speed IR, which is not sufficient for the 100 speed IR
Center detector selected	↑	Since the thoracic spine lies over the center detector, the spine has appropriate density, but the lungs have too much density.
70 kVp	0	Changing the kVp does not affect the density, because AEC simply waits for the right number of photons to exit the patient. However, the contrast is increased.
100 mA	0	Changing the mA does not affect the density, because AEC simply waits for the right number of photons to exit the patient. However, the length of exposure is increased.
−2 density	↓	Changing the density selector actually changes the setting of the AEC so it turns off the exposure much sooner, resulting in reduced density.
Selecting the table Bucky setting but still using the upright Bucky	↑	The AEC device in the table Bucky is waiting for enough exit radiation to hit so that the exposure can be terminated. Because the x-ray beam is aimed at the upright Bucky it is a very long exposure and results in increased density.
Patient has cardiac pacemaker positioned over detector	↑	The detector that is behind the pacemaker takes a long time to turn off the exposure because the radiation has to pass through the pacemaker. This results in increased density.

TABLE II-2   DIGITAL RADIOGRAPHY AND AEC

An upright PA chest exam is done as indicated above, except that now a CR system is used instead of film-screen.

Assuming all other factors remain the same, unless indicated, how would the following changes affect the density of the image?

Change	Effect on Density in Area of Interest	Explanation
CR image receptor	0	The AEC is calibrated to the 400 speed system. The exposure ends when the exposure is sufficient for the 400 speed IR, which is less than optimal for the 200 speed CR image receptor. The computer adjusts the density, but quantum mottle is apparent due to underexposure of the IP.
Center detector selected*	0	Since the thoracic spine lies over the center detector, the IP receives more exposure than is needed. The computer adjusts the density but the image contrast is reduced due to excessive scatter, and the patient is overexposed.
70 kVp*	0	The exposure to the IP remains the same and the computer adjusts for density. However, the contrast is increased due to the reduced kVp.
100 mA*	0	The exposure to the IP remains the same and the computer adjusts for density. However, the length of exposure is increased.
−2 density*	0	The exposure terminates much sooner, with one half the exposure to the IP. The computer adjusts the density, but quantum mottle is apparent due to underexposure of the IP.
Selecting the table Bucky setting but still using the upright Bucky*	0	Excessive radiation reaches the IP since the detectors in the table Bucky are unable to terminate the exposure. The computer adjusts the density but the image contrast is reduced due to excessive scatter, and the patient is overexposed.
Patient has cardiac pacemaker positioned over detector*	0	The detector that is behind the pacemaker takes a long time to turn the exposure off, since the radiation has to pass through the pacemaker. The computer adjusts the density but the image contrast is reduced due to excessive scatter, and the patient is overexposed.

*AEC is now calibrated for 200 speed system

FILM CRITIQUE

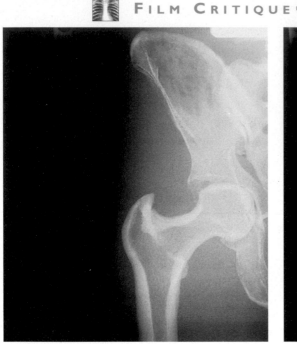 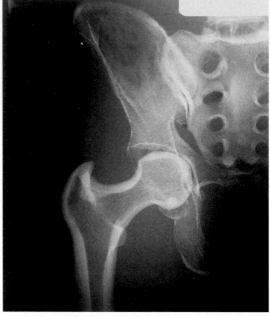

FIGURE 11-9 Image A is produced using 70 kVp, 200 mA, AEC exposure, center detector, 400 speed film-screen combination, and a 40-inch source-to-image receptor distance.

FIGURE 11-10 Image B is produced using 70 kVp, 200 mA, AEC exposure, center detector, 400 speed film-screen combination, and a 40-inch source-to-image receptor distance.

1. Evaluate each radiograph and discuss its quality (Figures 11-9 and 11-10).
2. For each image, evaluate its exposure variables and discuss their effect on the quality of the image (regardless of whether it is apparent on the radiograph).
3. For each image, identify any adjustments that could be made in the exposure factors to produce an optimal image.

1. The purpose of using AEC with film-screen imaging is to control
   A. kVp.
   B. mA.
   C. density.
   D. contrast.

2. AEC devices work by measuring
   A. radiation leaving the tube.
   B. radiation that exits the patient.
   C. radiation that is absorbed by the patient.
   D. attenuation of primary radiation by the patient.

3. How many detectors are typically found in an AEC system?
   A. 1
   B. 2
   C. 3
   D. 4

4. Minimum response time refers to
   A. the proper exposure time needed for an optimal exposure when an AEC device is used.
   B. exposure time minus the amount of time the AEC detectors are measuring radiation.
   C. the difference in exposure times between AEC systems and electronic timers.
   D. the shortest exposure time possible when an AEC device is used.

5. Which of the following statements about AEC with film-screen examinations is true?
   A. Adjusting the mA value affects image density.
   B. Adjusting the kVp value affects image density.
   C. Adjusting the backup time affects image density.
   D. Adjusting the density controls affects image density.

6. Which one of the following statements comparing ionization chamber AEC systems with photomultiplier (PM) tube systems is true?
   A. Ionization chamber systems are accurately called *phototimers*.
   B. Ionization chamber systems measure radiation before it interacts with the cassette.
   C. PM tube systems are more modern.
   D. PM tube systems measure radiation before it interacts with the cassette.

7. The purpose of the backup timer is to
   A. ensure a diagnostic exposure each time AEC is used.
   B. produce consistent levels of density on all radiographs.
   C. determine the exposure time that is used.
   D. limit unnecessary x-ray exposure.

8. What happens if AEC is activated for a stretcher chest study?
   A. An inappropriately short exposure occurs.
   B. An inappropriately long exposure occurs.
   C. An appropriate exposure probably occurs.
   D. Underexposure of the radiograph occurs.

9. The purpose of anatomic programming is to
   A. present the radiographer with a preselected set of exposure factors.
   B. override AEC when the radiographer has made a mistake in its use.
   C. determine which AEC detectors should be used for a particular examination.
   D. prevent overexposure and underexposure of radiographs, which sometimes happen when AEC is used.

10. Which one statement concerning both AEC and APR is true?
    A. The skilled use of both requires less knowledge of exposure factors on the part of the radiographer.
    B. The use of both requires the radiographer to be less responsible for accurate centering of the anatomic part.
    C. The individual judgment and discretion of the radiographer is still necessary when using these.
    D. The tasks involved with practicing radiography generally are made more difficult with these systems.

11. When using AEC with digital imaging systems, assuming all other factors are correct, selecting the center chamber on a PA chest results in:
    A. decreased density in the lung area
    B. increased density in the lung area
    C. appropriate density in the lung area
    D. increased quantum mottle in the image
    E. both C and D

12. When using AEC with digital imaging systems, assuming all other factors are correct, selecting the minus 2 density on a PA chest results in:
    A. decreased density in the lung area
    B. increased density in the lung area
    C. appropriate density in the lung area
    D. increased quantum mottle in the image
    E. both C and D

CHAPTER 12

Digital Imaging

KEY TERMS

digital imaging
dynamic range
postprocessing image enhancement
matrix
pixel

imaging plate (IP)
histogram
algorithms
window level
window width

Advancements in computer technology have made digital imaging a reality in diagnostic radiography. Although the terminology has not yet been standardized, **digital imaging** is defined as an image constructed from numerical data. Digital imaging is not new to the radiologic sciences . Since the introduction of computed tomography (CT) in the 1970s, digital imaging has become standard in several modalities, such as magnetic resonance imaging (MRI), nuclear medicine, and sonography. Each of these modalities has specialized equipment to create images that can be displayed, manipulated, and stored as digital or numerical data.

Further technological advancements have created the opportunity for digital imaging in diagnostic radiography. Advances in computer performance, high-resolution display monitors and high-speed electronic networks have made digital imaging an economical replacement for film-screen imaging.

Different processes are available to obtain digital images (Figure 12-1). Digital imaging includes film digitizers, digital fluoroscopy and digital radiography. Digital radiography refers to those methods that acquire the image by various types of image receptors, such as computed radiography, and direct readout digital radiography.

Although film digitizers were one of the first methods of creating digital images, they are not commonly used today. Processed radiographs were placed in a film

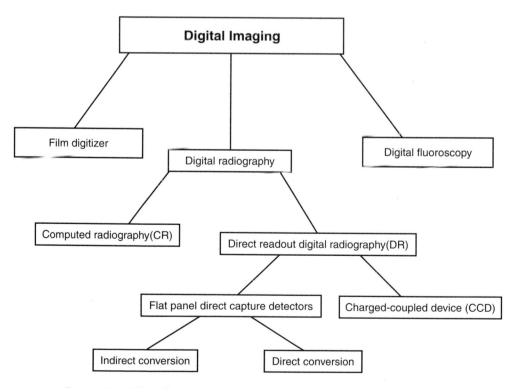

FIGURE 12-1 Digital imaging chart.

digitizer to convert the analog image into a digital image that could be sent electronically to a distant location. This method of creating a digital image resulted in an image with overall poor quality. Digital fluoroscopy and computed radiography have readily been introduced into radiology departments because of their compatibility with conventional x-ray equipment. Direct readout digital radiography cannot be easily used with existing conventional x-ray equipment and the radiographic system must be modified or replaced.

The value of digital imaging can be better understood by recognizing the limitations of conventional film-screen imaging.

Limitations of Conventional Imaging

The conventional film-screen system poses limitations that can be overcome in digital imaging. The radiographic image created following a divergent x-ray beam's attenuation results in the superimposition of anatomic structures. Obtaining multiple projections of an anatomic area will still result in overlying structures that obscure visualization of the area of interest.

Conventional radiography limits the visibility of a wide range of structures within the same anatomic part. An example is the difficulty of visualizing both soft tissue and bony structures within the same image. When an image is taken in the thorax region, the exposure technique must be selected depending on whether the area of interest is the lungs or the ribs. In addition, differentiation of soft tissue structures is limited because the attenuation of the x-ray beam among the soft tissues is so similar that the differences in visible densities (contrast) provide poor visualization.

A primary limiting factor of conventional radiography is that once the radiograph has been processed, the image is permanent and further adjustments cannot be made. If the image is considered to have excessive or insufficient density then it must be repeated, causing increased patient exposure.

The information displayed on the radiograph also is limited to the range of densities recorded on the film as a result of the absorption characteristics of the anatomic area. The radiograph does not provide any quantitative information about the attenuation characteristics of the anatomic tissues.

Processing time, storage, and archival of radiographs have created undesirable delays and costs. The amount of time it takes to process the film before viewing the radiograph can delay the progress of an examination or the diagnosis. In addition, the cost of storing radiographs and then retrieving them when needed for comparison has become unmanageable.

Digital imaging has overcome many of the limitations of conventional radiography. Radiographic images can be obtained, processed, stored, and retrieved in a more timely manner. The digital image has the ability to record a wider range of tissues with one exposure, provide quantitative data on the attenuation characteristics of the tissues, and visualize the anatomic area without overlying structures.

Digital Versus Conventional Imaging

Although digital imaging can overcome many of the limitations of conventional radiography, the two processes share several similarities.

SIMILARITIES

The radiographer continues to select the required exposure factors of milliamperage (mA), exposure time, and kilovoltage peak (kVp). In addition, accurate positioning of the patient for a variety of projections remains a critical part of the imaging process. Various accessory devices such as grids and collimators are still used for digital imaging. Regardless of the type, the image receptor receives the varying radiation intensities exiting the anatomic part. Although the image receptor is different, a latent image is still produced and processed to form a manifest image.

DIFFERENCES

The special features of digital imaging are significant in overcoming the limitations of conventional radiography.

The digital image receptor can respond to a wider range of x-ray exposures (wide dynamic range) than conventional film. The range of exposures a system can retain to create the visible image defines its **dynamic range**. The response of the image receptor in digital imaging is linear as opposed to curvilinear for radiographic film (Figure 12-2). As a result, the digital image can display a greater range of radiographic densities. After one x-ray exposure, anatomic areas having a wide range of composition such as soft tissues and bony structures can easily be visualized.

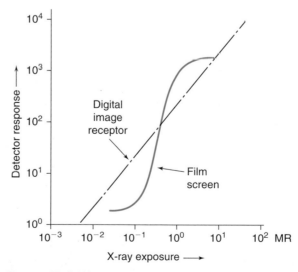

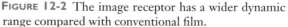

FIGURE 12-2 The image receptor has a wider dynamic range compared with conventional film.

An imaging system's dynamic range can be expressed numerically as a ratio. The greater the ratio, the greater the dynamic range. For example, film-screen systems have a dynamic range of 30:1, whereas, a digital system has a dynamic range greater than 1,000:1.

The digital image is composed of numerical data that can be easily manipulated by a computer. Once the image is converted into digital (numerical) data, the computer can perform **postprocessing image enhancement.** This process allows the manipulation of the image in a variety of ways, such as subtraction, contrast, and edge enhancement.

Digital Image Characteristics

Unlike a conventional radiograph that is made up of minute deposits of black metallic silver, a digital image is displayed as a combination of rows and columns that is called a **matrix.** The smallest component of the matrix is the **pixel** (picture element). The location of the pixel within the image matrix corresponds to an area within the patient or volume of tissue (Figure 12-3).

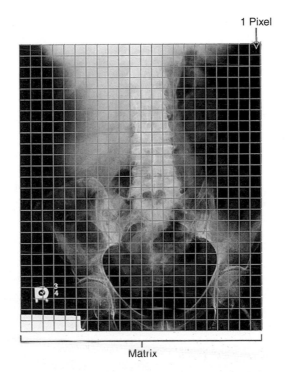

1 Pixel

Matrix

FIGURE 12-3 Location of the pixel within the image matrix corresponds to an area within the patient or volume of tissue.

For a given anatomic area (image size), a matrix size of 1024 × 1024 has 1,048,576 individual pixels, whereas a matrix size of 2048 × 2048 has 4,194,304 pixels. Image quality is improved with a larger matrix size that includes a greater number of smaller pixels (Figure 12-4 and Box 12-1).

A numeric value (bit) representing a shade of gray is stored for each pixel. This shade of gray is viewed as brightness on a cathode-ray-tube (CRT) or video monitor. "The brightness in each pixel is represented by a long list of digital numbers [digital

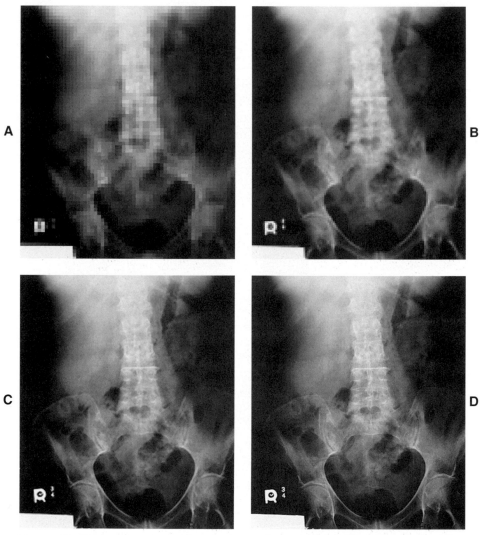

FIGURE 12-4 For a given image size, the larger the matrix size, the greater the number of smaller individual pixels. Increasing the number of pixels will improve the quality of the image. **A,** Matrix size is 64 × 64. **B,** Matrix size is 215 × 215. **C,** Matrix size is 1024 × 1024. **D,** Matrix size is 2048 × 2048.

code]; each number represents the intensity of a pixel, and the number's location in the list represents the pixel's location in the image."[1] (Figure 12-5) Each pixel has a bit depth and the number of bits determines the number of shades of gray the system is capable of displaying on the digital image. An 8-bit pixel can display 256 shades of gray, whereas a 10- and 12-bit pixel can display 1024 and 4096 shades of gray, respectively. A system that can display a greater number of shades of gray has better image quality.

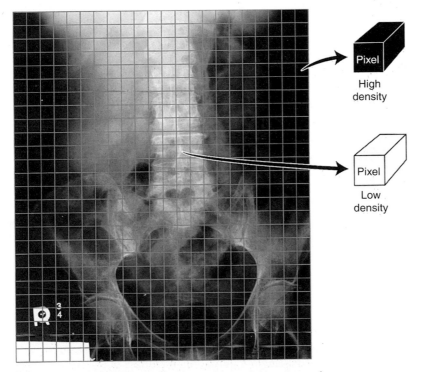

FIGURE 12-5 Each pixel represents a volume of tissue imaged.

[1]Kuni C: Introduction to computers & digital processing in medical imaging, Chicago, 1988, Year-Book Medical Publishers

Matrix Size and Image Quality

Increasing the matrix size increases the number of pixels, thereby increasing the quality of the image. Decreasing the matrix size decreases the number of pixels, thereby decreasing the quality of the image.

Digital Image Acquisition

Except for film digitizers and digital fluoroscopy, three primary stages are involved in digital imaging: image acquisition; image processing, and image display. During image acquisition, the type of image receptor used to receive the radiation exiting the anatomic area of interest characterizes each method. Once the exit radiation is converted to numerical (digital) data, image processing and display are the same, regardless of the methods used.

DIGITAL FLUOROSCOPY

Digital fluoroscopy has been introduced into the radiology department because it can readily be adapted to the image-intensification systems currently used. The fluoroscopic image is obtained in a manner similar to that of conventional fluoroscopy. The exit radiation is absorbed by the input phosphor, converted to electrons, sent to the output phosphor, released as visible light, and converted to a an electronic video signal for transmission to the television monitor.

In digital fluoroscopy (Figure 12-6), an analog-to-digital converter (ADC) is used to convert the analog (continuous) video signal to digital (numeric) data. The image is then viewed on a high-resolution video monitor. It is the conversion of the video signal to digital data that creates the opportunity for manipulation of the image in a variety of ways.

DIGITAL RADIOGRAPHY

Methods categorized as digital radiography are differentiated from film digitizers and digital fluoroscopy by the method of image acquisition. Computed radiography (CR) and Direct Readout Digital Radiography (DR) include a type of image receptor that receives the exit radiation and, by differing methods, converts the varying x-ray intensities into digital data.

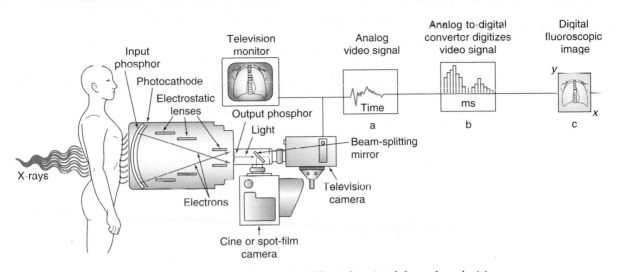

FIGURE 12-6 Analog and digital signals in fluoroscopy. The video signal from the television camera is analog, where the voltage signal varies continuously. This analog signal is sampled (*a*), producing a stepped representation of the analog video signal (*b*). The numerical values of each step are stored (*c*), producing a matrix of digital image data. The binary representation of each pixel value in the matrix is stored and can be manipulated by a computer. The value of each pixel can be mapped to a brightness level for viewing on a CRT or to an optical density for hard copy on film. *Image © Eastman Kodak Company.*

Computed Radiography (CR)

As introduced in Chapter 7, the radiation exiting the patient interacts with the **imaging plate (IP)**, where the photon intensities are absorbed by the photostimulable phosphor Figure 12-7). Although some of the absorbed energy is released as visible light (luminescence), as in conventional radiography, a sufficient amount of energy is stored in the phosphor to produce a latent image. The latent image is formed within the crystals of the photostimulable phosphor after the transfer of energy by the photoelectric effect.

Although the imaging plate can store the absorbed energy for several hours, the latent image must be processed in a timely manner or the stored energy will fade along with the latent image.

The exposed imaging plate is placed in a reader unit that converts the analog image into a digital image for computer processing (Figure 12-8). Units are available in single-plate and multiplate readers. Once in the reader unit, the imaging plate is scanned with a helium-neon laser beam to release the stored energy as visible light (Figure 12-9). A photomultiplier tube (PMT) collects, amplifies, and converts the light to an electrical signal proportional to the range of energies stored in the

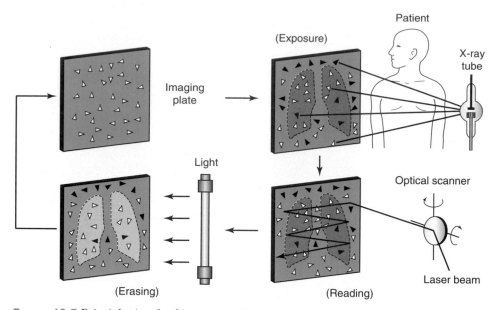

FIGURE 12-7 Principles involved in computed radiography. *Courtesy Fuji Medical Systems.*

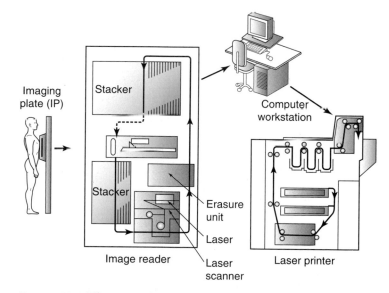

FIGURE 12-8 The exposed CR imaging plate is placed in a reader unit to release the stored image, convert the analog image to a digital image, and send the data to a computer monitor, laser printer, or both for a hard copy. The reader unit also erases the exposed imaging plate in preparation for the next exposure.

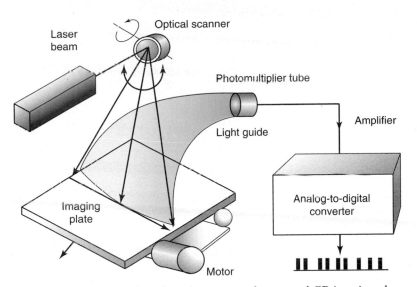

FIGURE 12-9 A neon-helium laser beam scans the exposed CR imaging plate to release the stored energy as visible light. The photomultiplier tube collects, amplifies, and converts the light to an electrical signal. The analog-to-digital converter converts the analog data to digital data.

imaging plate. The electrical signals are analyzed for comparison to preprogrammed information and altered according to the intensity of the exposure.

Before the imaging plate is stored for later use, the plate is scanned with an intense light to release any residual energy that could affect future exposures. Photostimulable phosphors can be reused and are estimated to have a life of 10,000 readings before they need to be replaced.

Manufacturers of computed radiography systems have different methods of indicating the x-ray exposure. Each type of system specifies the expected range of x-ray exposure sufficient to produce a quality image. A number is placed on the processed image to indicate the level of x-ray exposure received (incident exposure) to the imaging plate. Depending on the manufacturer of the system, the numerical indicator may be inversely proportional or directly proportional to the incident exposure. It is important for the radiographer to consider the indicated value because exposure errors affect the quality of the digital image. Exposure errors result in high or low electrical signals that are normalized to provide digital images with diagnostic density or brightness. Although computed radiography offers the advantage of correcting for exposure errors, image quality can be sacrificed. X-ray exposure errors of more or less than 50% may produce poor-quality images.

Advantages of CR are its compatibility with existing film-screen x-ray equipment and its use in mobile imaging. Disadvantages include the amount of time necessary for processing and image readout and the potential for increased x-ray exposures to achieve comparable image quality to film-screen methods.

Direct Readout Digital Radiography (DR)

Direct Readout Digital radiography (DR) involves the use of electronic x-ray detectors that receive the exit radiation and convert the varying x-ray intensities into electronic signals that are processed by a computer workstation. Electronic direct readout detectors are what differentiate DR from CR. Several types of electronic detectors are available for digital radiography.

Charged-coupled Device (CCD)

Charged-coupled device (CCD) is a fixed image receptor located at the site of the x-ray interactions. CCDs use a phosphor type screen (scintillator) to receive the exit radiation and convert them to varying light intensities; light sensitive electrodes then directly convert these light patterns to a digital signal. CCDs are physically small and require minification optics to image the light emitted by the scintillator. CCDs have not been widely used in digital radiography.

Flat Panel Direct Capture Systems

Flat panel digital systems are constructed so the large area detector and electronics are adjacent to the site of the x-ray interactions. The detector system is integrated and fixed in the table or upright Bucky system and therefore does not need to be transported for processing (Figure 12-10). Flat panel systems provide quicker access to better quality images when compared to film-screen and CR. Disadvantages include incompatiblity with existing x-ray equipment and inability to be used in mobile imaging.

Indirect Conversion Detectors

As introduced in Chapter 7, indirect conversion detectors use a scintillator to convert the exit radiation into visible light before the light is converted to an electronic charge. The electronic charge is stored in a thin-film transistor array before it is processed in the computer.

The design of the scintillator used to convert the x-ray intensities into visible light can be structured or unstructured. Structured scintillators, usually crystalline cesium iodide, reduce the spread of visible light and are considered to improve the quality of the digital image when compared with the unstructured type of scintillator. Indirect conversion detectors use a two-step process to convert x-ray intensities to visible light, and then the visible light is converted to electronic signals that represent the varying intensities. The electronic signals are then directed to amplifiers and an analog-to-digital converter (ADC) to produce the raw digital image.

Direct Conversion Detectors

Direct conversion detectors, as discussed in Chapter 7, use an amorphous selenium-coated detector to convert the exit radiation directly into electric charges. Similar to with indirect conversion detectors, the electronic charge is stored in a thin-film transistor array before it is directed to amplifiers and an analog-to-digital converter (ADC) and then processed in the computer.

It is anticipated that radiology departments will be designed to combine the use of both CR and DR imaging systems. Regardless of the type of digital imaging system,

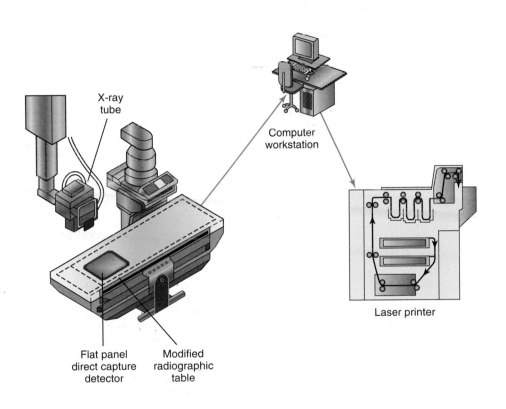

X-ray
tube

Computer
workstation

Laser printer

Flat panel
direct capture
detector

Modified
radiographic
table

FIGURE 12-10 Flat panel digital detector fixed in a modified x-ray table.

the varying electrical signals are sent to the ADC for conversion into digital data.
The digitized x-ray intensities or pixels are patterned in the computer to form the
image matrix. The image matrix is a digital composite of the varying x-ray intensities
exiting the patient. Each pixel has a brightness level representing the attenuation
characteristic of the volume of tissue imaged. Once the varying x-ray intensities are
converted to numerical data, the digital image can be processed, manipulated,
transported, or stored electronically. Figure 12-11 compares conventional and digital
radiographic methods of image acquisition. Table 12-1 compares the characteristics
of the different imaging methods.

Digital Image Processing

During image processing, the digital data are evaluated and manipulated before being
displayed. The digital data are used to construct a **histogram,** or graphic display, of

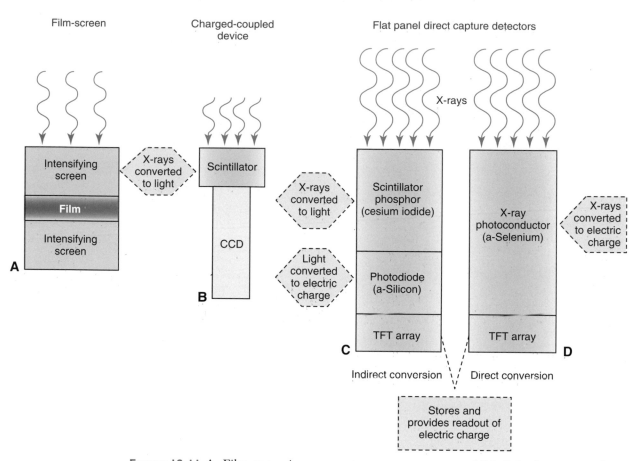

Film-screen

Charged-coupled device

Flat panel direct capture detectors

FIGURE 12-11 **A,** Film-screen image receptors convert x-rays to visible light that exposes the radiographic film. **B** and **C,** Detectors convert x-rays to visible light then to an electric charge. **D,** Direct conversion flat panel detectors convert the x-rays to electric signals.

the distribution of pixel values (Figure 12-12). Each image has its own histogram, and it is evaluated to determine the adequacy of the image receptor exposure to x-rays. If the histogram suggests a low or high exposure, the electrical signal will be adjusted accordingly to compensate for the error.

Processing **algorithms,** or mathematical formulas, are used to formulate image reconstruction for the specific type of examination performed, such as chest, extremity, spine, or abdomen. The radiographer must indicate the correct radiographic procedure so that the appropriate algorithm is performed. If the incorrect processing algorithm is selected, the resulting image is not reconstructed properly.

TABLE 12-1 COMPARING RADIOGRAPHIC IMAGING METHODS

Method	Image Receptor	Flexibility	Dynamic Range	Detective Quantum Efficiency (DQE)	System Relative Speed	Time to Image Viewing
Film-screen	Radiographic film and intensifying screen	Mobile	30:1	25%	400	~ 2 minutes
Computed Radiography (CR)	Photostimuable Phosphor Imaging Plate	Mobile	4,000:1	20-35%	200-300	~ 2 minutes
Flat Panel Direct Capture Systems (DR)	Indirect or Direct Conversion detectors	Fixed	10,000:1	65-70%	Faster than film-screen	~ 20 seconds

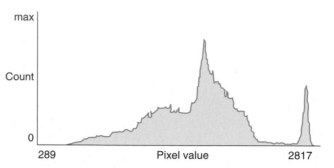

FIGURE 12-12 Histogram showing the number of each of the pixel values in an image. The pixel values (grays) are represented by the horizontal axis; the total number of each pixel value is reflected on the vertical axis. *From Cesar LJ: Computed radiography: its impact on radiographers, J ASRT 68(3), 1997.*

Digital Image Display

Once the image has been processed in a digital format, it can be displayed on a CRT, printed on film, sent to a distant location, or stored on a magnetic or optical disk.

CRT OR VIDEO MONITOR

When the computed image is displayed on a CRT (soft-copy viewing), it can be manipulated in a variety of ways. The following are four common postprocessing techniques:

1. *Subtraction* (Figure 12-13) is a technique that can remove superimposed structures so the anatomic area of interest is more visible. Because the image is in a digital format, the computer can subtract selected brightness values to create an image without superimposed structures.
2. *Contrast enhancement* (Figure 12-14) is a postprocessing technique that alters the pixel values to display different brightness levels.
3. *Edge enhancement* (Figure 12-15) is a postprocessing technique that improves the visibility of small, high-contrast structures.
4. *Black/white reversal* (Figure 12-16) is a postprocessing technique that reverses the gray scale from the original radiograph.

One of the factors that has limited the rapid introduction of digital imaging into radiology departments has been the display of images on a CRT. Standard monitors used in fluoroscopy have a 525-line system. Visualizing a digital image of similar quality to a conventional image requires that the display monitor have high spatial

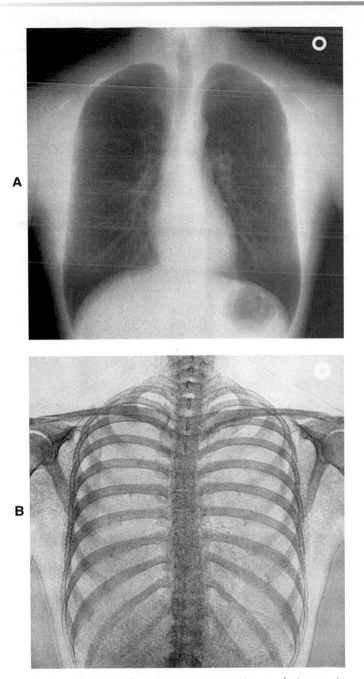

FIGURE 12-13 Subtraction postprocessing techniques. **A,** Skeletal areas are removed. **B,** Lungs and soft tissue are removed.

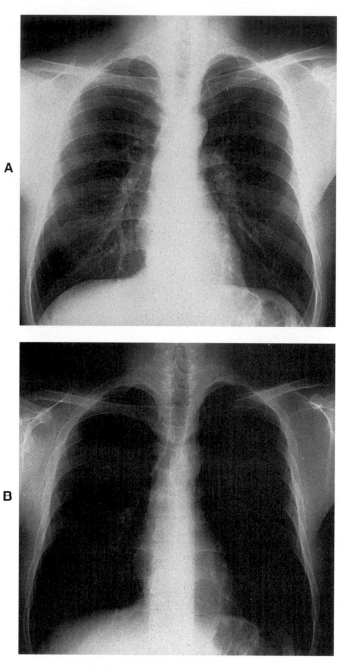

FIGURE 12-14 Postprocessing adjustment in radiographic contrast. **A,** Longer-scale contrast typical of chest radiography. **B,** Contrast has been adjusted to present a higher scale.

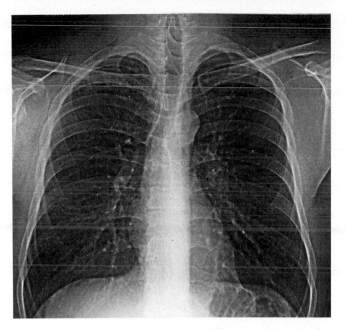

FIGURE 12-15 Radiographic image demonstrates an edge enhancement postprocessing technique.

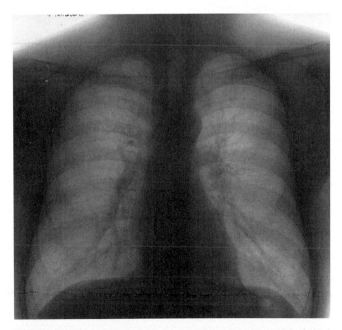

FIGURE 12-16 Radiographic image demonstrates a black and white reversal postprocessing technique.

resolution (recorded detail) capabilities. This can be achieved only with monitors that are at least 1000-line systems. The cost associated with installing high-resolution monitors in all locations that would benefit from this technology has been somewhat prohibitive.

LASER CAMERA PRINTING

As in conventional radiography, standard hard-copy viewing of images is still common. Digital images can be altered while being viewed on a CRT and then printed onto film by a laser camera. Multiple images can be printed on a single sheet, and multiple copies of images can be printed that were processed differently.

Laser printers are available that use either wet or dry printing methods. Wet laser printers use liquid chemicals in a developer and fixer to process the image. In dry processing the chemicals are part of the film. The image is created by use of heat instead of liquid chemicals.

Exposure Technique selection

The exposure technique should be selected based on the requirements for the type of radiographic procedure performed. Previous chapter discussions about manipulating the quantity and quality of the radiation, use of AEC and accessory devices, and controlling for scatter radiation all pertain to digital imaging.

What differentiates digital from film-screen imaging is the ability of the computer to adjust the density of the image for exposure technique errors. It should be noted that although the computer can adjust for both low- and high-exposure technique errors, the radiographer is still responsible for selecting exposure techniques that maintain patient exposure *As Low As Reasonably Achievable* (ALARA). In addition, exposure techniques that are too low adversely affect the quality of the image even though the computer can adjust the density. Exposure techniques selected that are too high result in excessive radiation exposure to the patient. It is recommended that radiographers continue to select exposure techniques that would produce optimal radiographic images, regardless of whether the imaging system is film-screen or digital.

Practical Tip

Exposure Technique Selection and Digital Imaging

Optimal exposure techniques should be selected regardless of whether film-screen or digital image receptors are used. Although the digital imaging system can adjust for exposure technique errors, poor image quality or increased radiation exposure to the patient may result.

Digital Image Quality

Detective Quantum Efficiency (DQE) is a term frequently associated with digital imaging. It is an objective measure that evaluates the overall efficiency of converting the information from x-ray intensities into a radiographic image. Digital systems can be rated according to their DQE and are usually stated as a percentage. A system that has a DQE of 100% is a (theoretically) perfect imaging system, but there are no perfect radiographic imaging systems. Direct Readout Digital Radiography systems have been said to have higher DQE when compared with other imaging systems. DQE is a complex method of evaluating and comparing image quality, and the methods for determining a system's performance should be comparable.

The following section on digital image quality is presented using terminology similar to film-screen image quality. Evaluating the quality of digital images shares many of the same properties as in conventional radiography. Resolution, density, and contrast are all attributes important in the production of quality radiographic images.

RESOLUTION

Spatial resolution is a characteristic of digital imaging comparable to the geometric properties of conventional radiographic imaging.

Although digital imaging technology has been available since the 1970s, a limiting factor has been its low spatial resolution. Recent improvements in image receptors and display monitors have contributed to the improved resolution of digital images. Transforming data of a continuous form (analog) to a discrete form (digital) results in the loss of some information. Conventional radiography has the capability of resolving approximately 6 to 10 Lp/mm (line pairs per millimeter), whereas computed radiography has been limited to approximately 2.5 to 5 Lp/mm. Resolution also is sacrificed during x-ray absorption by the photostimulable phosphor and laser scanning to extract the absorbed energy. Newer CR systems have improved the spatial resolution so it is more comparable with conventional radiography.

Flat panel direct capture detectors are said to have improved spatial resolution when compared with CR. The direct readout electronics reduce the loss of information noted with CR.

A major factor in the level of spatial resolution of digital images is the pixel size. As mentioned previously, the greater the number of pixels in a matrix image, the smaller their size. An image consisting of a greater number of pixels provides improved spatial resolution. Overall, spatial resolution is limited to the size of the pixel.

Important Relationship

Pixel Number and Spatial Resolution

Increasing the number of pixels in the image matrix increases the spatial resolution.

The capabilities of the device used for image viewing also affect the visibility of anatomic detail. As discussed, the CRT or video monitor has been a limiting factor in the widespread use of digital imaging. High-resolution monitors with 1000 lines have improved the image display. More recently, 2000-line resolution has been rcommended for CRT monitors that are used for diagnosis.

DENSITY

Visualizing anatomic structures within the area of interest on a conventional radiograph requires that the optical densities fall within the straight-line region of the sensitometric curve. When optical densities fall outside this region, the density is either excessive or insufficient, which usually necessitates a repeat study. Because digital imaging provides a wide dynamic range, the margin of error is greater for the exposure technique in obtaining densities that provide sufficient visualization of the anatomic area of interest.

The beam that exits the patient contains more than 1000 shades of gray. The visual range of the human eye is limited to about 32 shades of gray. The processed digital image is only a small sample of the total information contained within the computer.

The **window level** sets the midpoint of the range of densities visible in the image. Changing the window level on the CRT monitor allows the image brightness to be increased or dccrcased throughout the range of densities (Figure 12-17).

Adjusting the window level for image brightness on the CRT monitor has the opposite effect on the image density printed for a hard copy. Increasing the window level on the CRT image (increased brightness) decreases the density on the hard-copy film, whereas decreasing the window level on the CRT image (decreased brightness) increases density on the hard copy.

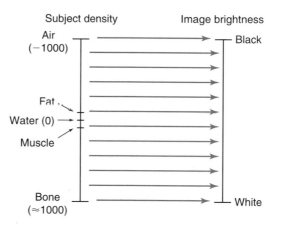

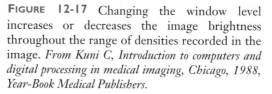

FIGURE 12-17 Changing the window level increases or decreases the image brightness throughout the range of densities recorded in the image. *From Kuni C, Introduction to computers and digital processing in medical imaging, Chicago, 1988, Year-Book Medical Publishers.*

Important Relationship

Window Level and Image Brightness

A direct relationship exists between window level and image brightness on the CRT monitor. Increasing the window level increases the image brightness; decreasing the window level decreases the image brightness.

CONTRAST

An important distinguishing characteristic of a digital image is its improved contrast resolution when compared to a film-screen image. The contrast resolution of the imaging system determines the level of visibility of small objects having similar densities or shades of gray. As mentioned previously, the depth of the pixel is determined by the number of bits (i.e. 8, 10 or 12), which affects the number of shades of gray available for image display. Increasing the number of shades of gray increases the contrast resolution within the image. An image with increased contrast resolution increases the visibility of recorded detail.

Important Relationship

Pixel Depth and Contrast Resolution

The greater the pixel depth (i.e. 12-bit) the greater the number of shades of gray available for image display. Increasing the number of shades of gray available to display on a digital image improves its contrast resolution.

Many of the same principles used to vary contrast in conventional radiography are applicable to digital imaging. Kilovoltage remains the primary exposure factor used to manipulate subject contrast. The kilovoltage should be selected based on the penetration needed, but more importantly, it should be selected to produce the level of contrast (high or low) necessary to best visualize the anatomic area of interest. Because the image receptors used in digital imaging are more sensitive to scatter radiation, efforts to reduce the amount of scatter radiation reaching the image receptor should be increased.

As discussed in Chapter 6, many of the factors used in conventional radiography to control or limit the amount of scatter radiation reaching the film are also used digital imaging. Grids typically are used with larger anatomic structures to limit the amount of scatter reaching the image receptor. In addition, appropriate collimation is used to reduce the amount of scatter interacting with the imaging receptor.

Once the digital image is processed, radiographic contrast can be adjusted to vary visualization of the area of interest. The **window width** is a control that adjusts the radiographic contrast (Figure 12-18). Because the digital image can display densities ranging from –1000 (black) to +1000 (white), the display monitor can vary the range or number of densities visible on the image. Adjusting the range of densities visible varies the scale of contrast. When the entire range of densities is displayed (wide window width), the image has lower contrast, or more shades of gray; when a smaller range of densities is displayed (narrow window width), the image has higher contrast, or fewer shades of gray (Figure 12-19).

This concept is similar to conventional radiography regarding scale of contrast. In conventional radiography, radiographic contrast is inversely related to the range of visible densities. A high-contrast radiograph (few shades of gray) displays a smaller (narrow) range of densities, whereas a lower-contrast radiograph (many shades of gray) displays a greater (wider) range of visible densities.

In digital imaging, an inverse relationship also exists between window width and image contrast.

Important Relationship

Window Width and Radiographic Contrast

A narrow (decreased) window width increases radiographic contrast, whereas a wider (increased) window width decreases radiographic contrast.

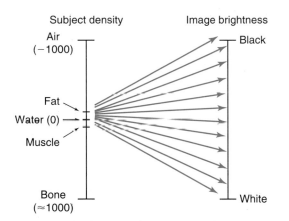

FIGURE 12-18 Changing the window width increases or decreases the range of densities visible. A narrow window width decreases the range of densities and increases contrast. Wider window width increases the range of densities and reduces contrast. *From Kuni C, Introduction to computers and digital processing in medical imaging, Chicago, 1988, Year-Book Medical Publishers.*

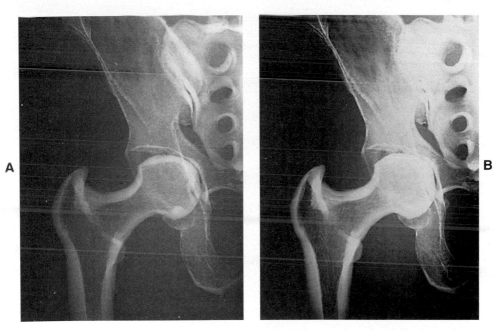

FIGURE 12-19 Changing the window width varies the scale of contrast visible on the computed image.

NOISE

Image noise contributes no useful diagnostic information and serves only to detract from the quality of the image. As in conventional radiography, quantum mottle is the primary source of noise in digital imaging and it is photon dependent. Quantum mottle is visible as density fluctuations on the image. The fewer photons reaching the image receptor to form the image, the greater the quantum mottle visible on the digital image.

Important Relationship

Number of Photons and Quantum Mottle

Decreasing the number of photons reaching the image receptor increases the amount of quantum mottle within the image; increasing the number of photons reaching the image receptor decreases the amount of quantum mottle within the image.

As mentioned previously, the digital system can adjust for low or high x-ray exposures during image acquisition. When the x-ray exposure to the image receptor is too low (decreased number of photons), the density can be corrected but the image displays increased quantum mottle or image noise (Figure 12-20).

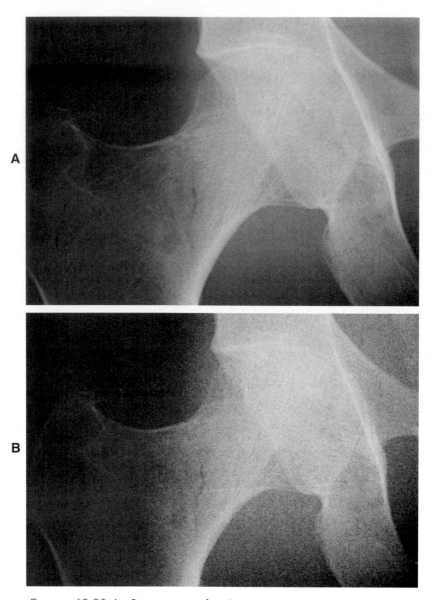

FIGURE 12-20 **A,** Image created using an appropriate x-ray exposure technique. **B,** Image demonstrates increased quantum mottle as a result of insufficient x-ray exposure to the image receptor.

Image noise contributes no useful information and only degrades the quality of the digital image. Image noise is more noticeable with the postprocessing techniques of contrast and edge enhancement.

The quality of the digital image depends on many of the same factors as conventional radiography. In addition to the effect of exposure factors, accurate positioning of the part and proper alignment of the part x-ray beam and image receptor also affect the quality of the image. The positioning and alignment factors have a greater effect on the quality of the image than in conventional radiography during manual exposure. Similar to when the automatic exposure control (AEC) is used, the resultant image can be adversely affected when the part is not positioned properly or not aligned to the correct photocell. "If the part, beam, and plate are misaligned in such a way that the exposure does not match the algorithm assumptions for that part, the data will not be properly processed to yield an image with expected density and contrast."[2]

Digital Communication Networks

Digital communication needs in radiology also include the processing and delivery of patient data and subsequent interpretation of radiologic procedures. The ability to integrate image, voice, and medical information simultaneously involves a more complex system. Picture archival and communication system (PACS) is the computer system for digital imaging; radiology information systems (RIS) and hospital information systems (HIS) are the computer systems for medical information. The ability to integrate these systems can be accomplished by networks. A network system links all of these computer systems so that images, patient data, and interpretations can be viewed simultaneously by people at different workstations (Figure 12-21). An important goal of a radiology network system is to provide the referring physician with the radiology report, patient data, and radiographic images at a convenient location and in a more timely manner.

The Digital Imaging and Communications in Medicine (DICOM) is a communication standard for information sharing between PACS and imaging modalities. The Health Level Seven standard (HL7) is a communication standard for medical information. Connectivity and communication among these systems is necessary for radiology to realize the full potential of digital communication. Network systems are currently being marketed to meet the demands in the radiation sciences.

[2]Burns C: Using computer digital radiography effectively, *Semin Radiol Tech* 1(1):24-36, 1993

Digital Communication Networks

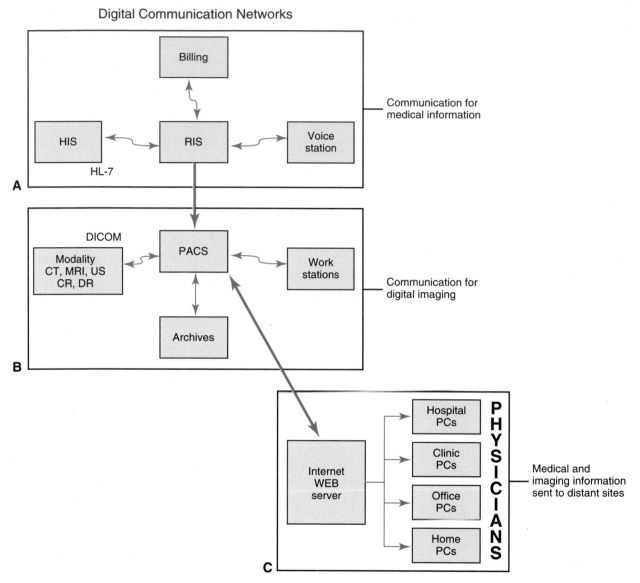

FIGURE 12-21 **A,** Communication among the computer systems for medical information. **B,** Communication among the computer systems for imaging. **C,** Referring physicians can receive radiology reports, patient data, and radiographic images through the Internet.

Review Questions

1. What is a limitation of conventional radiography?
   - **A.** Poor resolution
   - **B.** Poor soft tissue differentiation
   - **C.** Increased quantum mottle
   - **D.** Transporting cassettes

2. Computed radiography has the advantage of
   - **A.** less expensive equipment.
   - **B.** improved resolution.
   - **C.** latent image formation.
   - **D.** wide dynamic range.

3. What occurs when the exit radiation interacts with a photostimulable imaging plate?
   - **A.** Fluorescence
   - **B.** Energy absorption
   - **C.** Phosphorescence
   - **D.** Photoemission

4. A geometric characteristic of a computerized image is known as
   - **A.** sharpness.
   - **B.** noise.
   - **C.** mottle.
   - **D.** spatial resolution.

5. Image brightness on a CRT is adjusted by
   - **A.** scanning lines.
   - **B.** window level.
   - **C.** window width.
   - **D.** matrix size.

6. Radiographic contrast on a CRT is adjusted by
   - **A.** scanning lines.
   - **B.** window level.
   - **C.** window width.
   - **D.** matrix size.

7. Image noise can be decreased by
   - **A.** decreasing x-ray dose
   - **B.** increasing edge enhancement
   - **C.** increasing x-ray dose
   - **D.** decreasing window level

8. Increasing the window width of a digital image on a CRT
   - **A.** decreases the brightness.
   - **B.** increases the brightness.
   - **C.** decreases the contrast.
   - **D.** increases the contrast.

9. The smallest component of a matrix image that represents an x-ray intensity is called a(n)
   - **A.** pixel.
   - **B.** histogram.
   - **C.** algorithm.
   - **D.** brightness.

10. The mathematical formula used to construct a digital image is called a(n)
    - **A.** histogram.
    - **B.** algorithm.
    - **C.** postprocessing enhancement.
    - **D.** matrix.

11. Digital radiography includes image acquisition methods that include
    - **A.** computed radiography.
    - **B.** flat panel direct capture detectors.
    - **C.** charged-coupled devices.
    - **D.** all of the above.

12. A disadvantage of flat panel direct capture detectors is
    - **A.** increased patient dose.
    - **B.** cannot be used in mobile imaging.
    - **C.** increases time to view image.
    - **D.** narrow dynamic range.

Summary of Important Relationships

CHAPTER 1: RADIATION AND ITS DISCOVERY

The Dual Nature of X-Ray Energy

X-rays act both like waves and like particles. (See p. 6)

Wavelength and Frequency

Wavelength and frequency are inversely related. If one increases, the other decreases. (See p. 7)

CHAPTER 2: THE X-RAY BEAM

The Filament

The filament is the source of electrons during x-ray production. (See p. 15)

The Target

The target is the part of the anode that is struck by the focused stream of electrons coming from the cathode. The target stops the electrons and thus creates the opportunity for the production of x rays. (See p. 16)

Tungsten

Because tungsten has a high atomic number (74) and a high melting point (3370° F), it efficiently produces x-rays. (See p. 16)

Dissipating Heat

As heat is produced when the x-ray exposure is made, the rotating anode conducts the heat to the insulating oil that surrounds the x-ray tube. (See p. 17)

Rotating Anodes

Rotating anodes can withstand higher heat loads than stationary anodes because the rotation causes a greater physical area, or focal track, to be exposed to electrons. (See p. 18)

The Production of X-Rays

As electrons strike the target, their kinetic energy is transferred to the tungsten atoms in the anode to produce x-rays. (See p. 20)

Interactions That Produce X-Ray Photons

Bremsstrahlung interactions and characteristic interactions both produce x-ray photons. (See p. 20)

Bremsstrahlung Interactions

Most x-ray interactions in the diagnostic energy range are bremsstrahlung. (See p. 20)

Thermionic Emission

When the tungsten filament gains enough heat *(therm)*, the outer-shell electrons *(ions)* of the filament atoms are boiled off, or *emitted*, from the filament. (See p. 24)

Tube Current

Electrons flow in only one direction in the x-ray tube—from cathode to anode. This flow of electrons is called the *tube current* and is measured in milliamperes (mA). (See p. 26)

Energy Conversion in the X-Ray Tube

As electrons strike the anode target, approximately 99% of their kinetic energy is converted to heat, whereas only 1% (approximately) of their energy is converted to x-rays. (See p. 26)

Kilovoltage and the Speed of Electrons

The speed of the electrons traveling from the cathode to the anode increases as the kilovoltage applied across the x-ray tube increases. (See p. 28)

The Speed of Electrons and the Quality of the X-Rays

The speed of the electrons in the tube current determines the quality or energy of the x-rays that are produced. The quality or energy of the x-rays that are produced determines the penetrability of the primary beam. (See p. 28)

kVp and Beam Penetrability

As kVp increases, beam penetrability increases; as kVp decreases, beam penetrability decreases. (See p. 28)

Milliamperage, Tube Current, and X-Ray Quantity

The quantity of electrons in the tube current and quantity of x-rays produced are directly proportional to the milliamperage. (See p. 30)

Exposure Time, Tube Current, and X-Ray Quantity

The quantity of electrons that flows from cathode to anode and the quantity of x-rays produced are directly proportional to the exposure time. (See p. 31)

The Quantity of Electrons, X-Rays, and mAs

The quantity of electrons flowing from the cathode to the anode and the quantity of x-rays produced are directly proportional to mAs. (See p. 32)

Line Focus Principle

The line focus principle describes the relationship between the actual focal spot, where the electrons in the tube current bombard the target, and the effective focal spot, that same area as seen from directly below the tube. (See p. 32)

Anode Angle and Effective Focal Spot Size

Based on the line focus principle, the smaller the anode angle, the smaller the effective focal spot size. (See p. 33).

The Anode Heel Effect

X-rays are more intense on the cathode side of the tube. The intensity of the x-rays decreases toward the anode side. (See p. 34)

Low-Energy Photons, Patient Dose, and Image Formation

Low-energy photons serve only to increase patient dose and do not contribute to image formation. (See p. 36)

Heat Units

The number of HUs produced depends on the type of x-ray generator used and the exposure factors selected. (See p. 38)

CHAPTER 3: RADIOGRAPHIC IMAGE FORMATION

Differential Absorption and Image Formation

A radiographic image is created by passing an x-ray beam through the patient and interacting with an image receptor, such as a film-screen system. The variations in absorption and transmission of the exiting x-ray beam will structurally represent the anatomic area of interest. (See p. 47)

X-Ray Photon Absorption

During attenuation of the x-ray beam, the photoelectric effect is responsible for total absorption of the incoming x-ray photon. (See p. 47)

X-Ray Beam Scattering

During attenuation of the x-ray beam, the incoming x-ray photon may lose energy and change direction as a result of the Compton effect. (See p. 49)

Image Densities

The range of image densities is created by the variation in x-ray absorption and transmission as the x-ray beam passes through anatomic tissues. (See p. 51)

Fluoroscopy

Dynamic imaging of internal anatomic structures can be visualized with the use of an image intensifier. The exit radiation is absorbed by the input phosphor, converted to electrions, sent to the output phosphor, released as visible light, and then converted to an electronic video signal for transmission to the television monitor. (See p. 54)

Digital Imaging

The process of differential absorption for image formation remains the same for digital imaging. The varying x-ray intensities exiting the anatomic area of interest form the latent image. In digital imaging the latent image is stored as digital data and must be processed by the computer for viewing. (See p. 54)

CHAPTER 4: RADIOGRAPHIC IMAGE QUALITY: PHOTOGRAPHIC PROPERTIES

mAs, Quantity of Radiation, and Radiographic Density

As the mAs is increased, the amount of radiation is increased and radiographic density is increased. As the mAs is decreased, the amount of radiation is decreased and radiographic density is decreased. (See p. 61)

Milliamperage and Exposure Time

Milliamperage and exposure time have an inverse relationship when maintaining the same mAs. (See p. 62)

Kilovoltage and Radiographic Density

Increasing the kilovoltage peak increases the quantity of radiation reaching the image receptor and therefore increases radiographic density. Decreasing the kilovoltage peak decreases the quantity of radiation reaching the image receptor and therefore decreases radiographic density. (See p. 64)

SID and X-Ray Beam Intensity

As SID increases, the x-ray beam intensity is spread over a larger area. This decreases the overall intensity of the x-ray beam reaching the image receptor. (See p. 68)

SID and Radiographic Density

As SID increases, radiographic density decreases as a result of the square of the distance. As SID decreases, the radiographic density increases as a result of the square of the distance. (See p. 68)

SID and mAs

Increasing the SID requires that mAs be increased to maintain density, and decreasing the SID requires a decrease in mAs to maintain density. (See p. 68)

Grids and Radiographic Density

Adding, removing, or changing a grid requires an adjustment in mAs to maintain radiographic density. (See p. 70)

Film-Screen System Speed and Radiographic Density

The greater the speed of the film-screen system, the greater the amount of density produced on the radiograph; the lower the speed of the film-screen system, the less density produced on the radiograph. (See p. 71)

Film-Screen System Speed and mAs

Increasing the film-screen speed requires a decrease in the mAs to maintain density. Decreasing the film-screen speed requires an increase in the mAs to maintain density. (See p. 71)

Part Thickness and Radiographic Density

A thick anatomic part decreases the radiographic density. A thin anatomic part increases radiographic density. (See p. 73)

Exposure Factors and Digital Imaging

The relationship among the exposure factors of mAs, kVp and SID and their effect on the intensity of radiation reaching the image receptor holds true for digital imaging. (See p. 76)

Kilovoltage and Radiographic Contrast

High kilovoltage creates more densities but with fewer differences, resulting in a low-contrast (long-scale) image. Low kilovoltage creates fewer densities but with greater differences, resulting in a high-contrast (short-scale) image. (See p. 80)

Kilovoltage, Scatter Radiation, and Radiographic Contrast

Increasing kilovoltage increases the amount of scatter radiation produced and decreases radiographic contrast. Decreasing the kilovoltage decreases scatter production and reduces the amount of fog, therefore increasing radiographic contrast. (See p. 80)

Collimation and Radiographic Density

Increasing collimation (smaller field size) decreases radiographic density; decreasing collimation (wider field size) increases radiographic density. (See p. 82)

Scatter Radiation and Radiographic Contrast

Whenever the amount of scatter radiation reaching the image receptor is reduced, the radiographic contrast is increased (higher contrast). (See p. 82)

Part Thickness and Radiographic Contrast

Increasing part thickness lowers radiographic contrast because of more scatter radiation reaching the image receptor; decreasing part thickness increases radiographic contrast because of less scatter radiation reaching the image receptor. (See p. 84)

Scatter Radiation and Digital Imaging

Digital imaging receptors are more sensitive to scatter radiation than film-screen receptors. Efforts must be routinely made to limit the amount of scatter radiation reaching the digital image receptor. (See p. 87)

CHAPTER 5: RADIOGRAPHIC IMAGE QUALITY: GEOMETRIC PROPERTIES

Focal Spot Size and Recorded Detail

As focal spot size increases, unsharpness increases and recorded detail decreases; as focal spot size decreases, unsharpness decreases and recorded detail increases. (See p. 104)

SID, Unsharpness, and Recorded Detail

Increasing the SID decreases the amount of unsharpness and increases the amount of recorded detail in the image, whereas decreasing the SID increases the amount of unsharpness and decreases the recorded detail. (See p. 106)

OID, Unsharpness, and Recorded Detail

Increasing the OID increases the amount of unsharpness and decreases the recorded detail, whereas decreasing the amount of OID decreases the amount of unsharpness and increases the recorded detail. (See p. 107)

Intensifying Film-Screen Speed, Recorded Detail, and Unsharpness

Increasing the relative speed of the intensifying film-screen system decreases the recorded detail and increases the amount of unsharpness recorded in the image. Decreasing the relative speed of the intensifying film-screen system increases the recorded detail and decreases the amount of unsharpness recorded in the image. (See p. 109)

Motion and Recorded Detail

Motion of the tube, patient, part, or image receptor greatly decreases recorded detail. (See p. 112)

OID and Size Distortion

As OID increases, size distortion (magnification) increases; as OID decreases, size distortion (magnification) decreases. (See p. 114)

SID and Size Distortion

As SID increases, size distortion (magnification) decreases; as SID decreases, size distortion (magnification) increases. (See p. 115)

CHAPTER 6: SCATTER CONTROL

KVp and Scatter

The amount of scatter produced within the patient depends, in part, on the kVp selected. Exams using higher kVp's produce a greater proportion of scattered x-rays as compared to low kVp exams. (See p. 128)

X-ray Beam Field Size, Thickness of the Part, and Scatter

The larger the x-ray beam field size, the greater the amount of scatter radiation produced. The thicker the part being imaged, the greater the amount of scatter radiation produced. (See p. 128)

Volume of Tissue Irradiated and Scatter

The volume of tissue irradiated is affected by both the part thickness and the x-ray beam field size. Therefore the greater the volume of tissue irradiated, because of either or both factors, the greater the amount of scatter radiation produced. (See p. 129)

Beam Restriction and Patient Dose

As beam restriction or collimation increases, field size decreases and patient dose decreases. As beam restriction or collimation decreases, field size increases and patient dose increases. (See p. 129)

Collimation and Scatter Radiation

As collimation increases, the field size decreases and the quantity of scatter radiation decreases; as collimation decreases, the field size increases and the quantity of scatter radiation increases. (See p. 131)

Collimation and Radiographic Contrast

As collimation increases, the quantity of scatter radiation decreases, and radiographic contrast increases; as collimation decreases, the quantity of scatter radiation increases, and radiographic contrast decreases. (See p. 131)

Collimation and Radiographic Density

As collimation increases, radiographic density decreases; as collimation decreases, radiographic density increases. (See p. 132)

Scatter Radiation and Image Quality

Scatter radiation adds unwanted density to the radiograph and decreases image quality. (See p. 140)

Grid Ratio and Radiographic Contrast

As grid ratio increases, scatter cleanup improves and radiographic contrast increases; as grid ratio decreases, scatter cleanup is less effective and radiographic contrast decreases. (See p. 141)

Focused versus Parallel Grids

Focused grids have lead lines that are angled to approximately match the divergence of the primary beam. Thus focused grids allow more transmitted photons to reach the image receptor than parallel grids. (See p. 144)

Grid Ratio and Radiographic Density

As grid ratio increases, radiographic density decreases; as grid ratio decreases, radiographic density increases. (See p. 146)

Grid Ratio and Patient Dose

As grid ratio increases, patient dose increases; as grid ratio decreases, patient dose decreases. (See p. 149)

Upside-Down Focused Grids and Grid Cutoff

Placing a focused grid upside down on the image receptor causes the lateral edges of the radiograph to be very light (underexposed). (See p. 150)

Off-Level Error and Grid Cutoff

Angling the x-ray tube across the grid lines or angling the grid itself during exposure produces an overall decrease in density on the radiograph. (See p. 151)

Off-Center Error and Grid Cutoff

If the center of the x-ray beam is not aligned from side to side with the center of a focused grid, grid cutoff will occur. (See p. 152)

Off-Focus Error and Grid Cutoff

Using an SID outside of the focal range creates a loss of density at the periphery of the radiograph. (See p. 154)

Air Gap Technique and Scatter Control

The air gap technique is an alternative to using a grid to control scatter reaching the image receptor. By moving the image receptor away from the patient, more of the scatter radiation will miss the IR. The greater the gap, the less scatter reaches the IR. (See p. 156)

Digital Imaging and Scatter Control

Digital imaging systems are very sensitive to scatter radiation, as well as to overexposure and underexposure that results from grid cutoff and failure to make adjustments in mAs when needed. All of these factors result in reduced image quality. (See p. 157)

CHAPTER 7: IMAGE RECEPTORS

Sensitivity Specks and Latent Image Centers

Sensitivity specks serve as the focal point for the development of latent image centers. After exposure, these specks trap the free electrons and then attract and neutralize the positive silver ions. After enough silver is neutralized, the specks become a latent image center and are converted to black metallic silver after chemical processing. (See p. 167)

Silver Halide and Film Sensitivity

As the number of silver halide crystals increases, film sensitivity or speed increases; as the size of the silver halide crystals increases, film sensitivity or speed increases. (See p. 169)

Film Speed and Radiation Exposure

The faster the speed of a film, the less radiation exposure needed to produce a specific density. (See p. 169)

Spectral Matching and Density

To best use a film-screen system, the radiographer must match the color sensitivity of the film with the color emission of the intensifying screen. Failure to do so results in suboptimal density. (See p. 171)

Crossover and Recorded Detail

When light from one intensifying screen crosses over the film base and exposes the emulsion on the opposite side, loss of recorded detail occurs. Reducing crossover improves recorded detail. (See p. 172)

Screens, Patient Exposure, and Recorded Detail

Compared with direct-exposure radiography, adding intensifying screens reduces patient exposure but also reduces recorded detail. (See p. 173)

Screen Speed and Light Emission

The faster an intensifying screen, the more light emitted for the same intensity of x-ray exposure. (See p. 176)

Screen Speed and Patient Dose

As screen speed increases, less radiation is necessary and radiation dose to the patient decreases; as screen speed decreases, more radiation is necessary and radiation dose to the patient increases. (See p. 177)

Screen Speed and Density

For the same exposure, as screen speed increases, density increases; as screen speed decreases, density decreases. (See p. 177)

Rare Earth Phosphors and Speed

Rare earth phosphors are significantly faster than calcium tungstate because of increased absorption and conversion efficiency. (See p. 179)

Phosphor Thickness, Crystal Size, and Screen Speed

As the thickness of the phosphor layer increases, the speed of the intensifying screen increases; as the size of the phosphor crystals increases, the speed of the screen increases. (See p. 180)

Screen Speed and Recorded Detail

With any given phosphor type, as screen speed increases, recorded detail decreases, and as screen speed decreases, recorded detail increases. (See p. 182)

Latent Image Formation and Image Receptors

Latent image formation differs significantly among the three types of image receptors discussed in this chapter. Film's latent image is the result of deposits of silver ions at the sensitivity specks in the emulsion. CRs latent image is formed by electrons trapped in the barium fluorohalide crystals (in the phosphor layer). The latent image from direct-readout image receptors is the electric charge stored in the transistor. (See p. 188)

Chapter 8: Radiographic Film Processing

Producing Radiographic Densities

The developing agents are responsible for reducing the exposed silver halide crystals to metallic silver, visualized as optical densities. Phenidone is responsible for creating the lower densities, and hydroquinone is responsible for creating the higher densities. Their combined effect results in the range of visible densities on the radiograph. (See p. 198)

Clearing the Unexposed Crystals

The fixing agent, ammonium thiosulfate, is responsible for removing the unexposed crystals from the emulsion. (See p. 200)

Archival Quality of Radiographs

Maintaining the archival (long-term) quality of radiographs requires that most of the fixing agent be removed (washed) from the film. Staining or fading of the permanent image results when too much thiosulfate remains on the film. (See p. 201)

Archival Quality of Radiographs

Permanent radiographs must retain moisture of 10% to 15% to maintain archival quality. Excessive drying can cause the emulsion(s) to crack. (See p. 202)

Replenishment and Solution Performance

The replenishment system provides fresh chemicals to the developing and fixing solutions to maintain their chemical activity and volume when they become depleted during processing. (See p. 207)

Recirculation and Solution Performance

Recirculation of the developer and fixer solutions is necessary to maintain solution activity and the required agitation. (See p. 210)

Developer Temperature and Radiographic Quality

Variations in developer temperature adversely affect the quality of the radiographic image. Increasing developer temperature increases the density, and decreasing developer temperature decreases the density. Radiographic contrast also may be adversely affected by changes in the developer temperature. (See p. 212)

Moisture and Archival Quality

The dryer assembly controls the amount of moisture removal to maintain the archival quality of radiographic film. (See p. 214)

CHAPTER 9: SENSITOMETRY

Light Transmittance and Optical Density

As the percentage of light transmitted decreases, the optical density increases; as the percentage of light transmitted increases, the optical density decreases. (See p. 231)

Optical Density and Light Transmittance

For every 0.3 change in optical density, the percentage of light transmitted has changed by a factor of 2. A 0.3 increase in optical density results from a decrease in the percentage of light transmitted by half, whereas a 0.3 decrease in optical density results from an increase in the percentage of light transmitted by a factor of 2. (See p. 233)

Log Relative Exposure

A 0.3 change in log of exposure represents a change in intensity of radiation exposure by a factor of 2. An increase of 0.3 log of exposure results in a doubling of the amount of radiation exposure, whereas a decrease in 0.3 log of exposure results in halving the amount of radiation exposure. (See p. 235)

Film Speed and Optical Density

For a given exposure, as the speed of a film increases, the optical density produced also increases; as the speed of a film decreases, the optical density decreases. (See p. 237)

Film Speed and Speed Exposure Point

The lower the speed exposure point, the faster the film speed; the higher the speed exposure point, the slower the film speed. (See p. 238)

Slope and Film Contrast

The steeper the slope of the straight-line region (more vertical), the higher the film contrast; the lesser the slope (less vertical), the lower the film contrast. (See p. 241)

Average Gradient and Film Contrast

The greater the average gradient, the higher the film contrast; the lower the average gradient, the lower the film contrast. (See p. 243)

Exposure Latitude and Film Contrast

Exposure latitude and film contrast have an inverse relationship. High-contrast radiographic film has narrow latitude, and low-contrast film has wide latitude. (See p. 244)

CHAPTER 10: EXPOSURE FACTOR SELECTION

Exposure Technique Charts and Radiographic Quality

A properly designed and used technique chart standardizes the selection of exposure factors to help the radiographer produce consistent quality radiographs while minimizing patient exposure. (See p. 254)

Variable kVp/Fixed mAs Technique Chart

The variable kVp chart adjusts the kVp for changes in part thickness while maintaining a fixed mAs. (See p. 258)

Fixed kVp/Variable mAs Technique Charts

Fixed kVp/variable mAs technique charts identify optimal kVp values and alter the mAs for variations in part thickness. (See p. 260)

CHAPTER 11: AUTOMATIC EXPOSURE CONTROL

X-Ray Exposure and Density

The amount of density on a film depends on the amount of radiation exposure reaching the film. The greater the exposure to the film, the greater the resulting density. (See p. 268)

Principle of AEC Operation

Once a predetermined amount of radiation is transmitted through a patient, the x-ray exposure is terminated. This determines the exposure time and therefore the resulting density. (See p. 270)

Radiation-Measuring Devices

Detectors are the AEC devices that measure the amount of radiation transmitted. The radiographer selects which of the three detectors to use. (See p. 270)

Function of the Ionization Chamber

The ionization chamber interacts with exit radiation before it reaches the image receptor. Air in the chamber is ionized, and an electric charge that is proportional to the amount of radiation is created. (See p. 272)

Accurate Part Centering and Detector Selection

Accurate centering and detector selection are critical with AEC systems because the radiograph will demonstrate optimal density of the anatomy located directly over the detector. If the area of radiographic interest is not directly over the selected detector, that area probably will be overexposed or underexposed. (See p. 274)

Function of Backup Time

Backup time, the maximum exposure time allowed during an AEC examination, serves as a safety mechanism when the AEC is not used or is not functioning properly. (See p. 278)

Setting Backup Time

Backup time should be set at 150% to 200% of the expected exposure time. This allows the properly used AEC system to appropriately terminate the exposure but protects the patient and tube from excessive exposure if a problem occurs. (See p. 278)

The Patient and AEC

If the anatomic area directly over the detector does not represent the anatomic area of interest, inappropriate density may result. This can happen when the anatomic area over the detector contains a foreign object, a pocket of air, or contrast media, or if the anatomic area does not completely cover the detector. (See p. 279)

AEC and Digital Radiography

The radiographer must use AEC accurately when using digital imaging systems. Failure to do so can result in overexposure of the patient to ionizing radiation or production of an image that is of poor quality. (See p. 283)

CHAPTER 12: DIGITAL IMAGING

Matrix Size and Image Quality

Increasing the matrix size increases the number of pixels, thereby increasing the quality of the image. Decreasing the matrix size decreases the number of pixels, thereby decreasing the quality of the image. (See p. 298)

Pixel Number and Spatial Resolution

Increasing the number of pixels in the image matrix increases the spatial resolution. (See p. 311)

Window Level and Image Brightness

A direct relationship exists between window level and image brightness on the CRT monitor. Increasing the window level increases the image brightness; decreasing the window level decreases the image brightness. (See p. 313)

Pixel Depth and Contrast Resolution

The greater the pixel depth (i.e. 12-bit) the greater the number of shades of gray available for image display. Increasing the number of shades of gray available to display on a digital image improves its contrast resolution. (See p. 313)

Window Width and Radiographic Contrast

A narrow (decreased) window width increases radiographic contrast, whereas a wider (increased) window width decreases radiographic contrast. (See p. 314)

Number of Photons and Quantum Mottle

Decreasing the number of photons reaching the image receptor increases the amount of quantum mottle within the image; increasing the number of photons reaching the image receptor decreases the amount of quantum mottle within the image. (See p. 315)

Summary of Mathematical Applications

CHAPTER 2: THE X-RAY BEAM

Calculating mAs

$$mAs = mA \times seconds$$

Examples:

200 mA × .25 s   = 50 mAs

500 mA × 2/5 s   = 200 mAs

800 mA × 100 ms (milliseconds) = 80 mAs

(See p. 31)

Calculating Heat Units

An exposure is made with a three phase, 12 pulse x-ray unit using 600 mA, and 0.05 seconds, 75 kVp. How many heat units are produced from this exposure?

$$HU = mA \times time \times kVp \times generator\ factor$$
$$HU = 600 \times 0.05 \times 75 \times 1.41$$
$$= 3172.5\ HU$$

(See p. 38-39)

CHAPTER 4: RADIOGRAPHIC IMAGE QUALITY: PHOTOGRAPHIC PROPERTIES

Adjusting Milliamperage or Exposure Time

100 mA @ 0.10 s = 10 mAs. To increase the mAs to 20, you could use:

200 mA @ 0.10 s = 20 mAs

100 mA @ 0.20 s = 20 mAs

(See p. 61)

Adjusting Milliamperage and Exposure Time to maintain mAs

100 mA @ 100 ms (0.10 s) = 10 mAs. To maintain the mAs, you could use:

$$200 \text{ mA @ } 50 \text{ ms } (0.05 \text{ s}) = 10 \text{ mAs}$$
$$50 \text{ mA @ } 200 \text{ ms } (0.20 \text{ s}) = 10 \text{ mAs}$$

(See p. 62)

Using the 15% Rule

To increase density: Multiply the kVp by 1.15 (original kVp + 15%).

$$80 \text{ kVp} \times 1.15 = 92 \text{ kVp}$$

To decrease density: Multiply the kVp by 0.85 (original kVp − 15%).

$$80 \text{ kVp} \times 0.85 = 68 \text{ kVp}$$

To maintain density:

When increasing kVp by 15% (kVp × 1.15), divide the original mAs by 2.

$$80 \text{ kVp} \times 1.15 = 92 \text{ kVp and mAs}/2$$

When decreasing the kVp by 15% (kVp × 0.85), multiply the mAs by 2.

$$80 \text{ kVp} \times 0.85 = 68 \text{ kVp and mAs} \times 2$$

(See p. 66)

Inverse Square Law Formula

$$\frac{I_1}{I_2} = \frac{(D_2)^2}{(D_1)^2}$$

The intensity of radiation at an SID of 40 inches is equal to 500 mR. What is the intensity of radiation when the distance is increased to 56 inches?

$$\frac{500 \text{ mR}}{X} = \frac{(56)^2}{(40)^2}$$

$$500 \text{ mR} \times 1600 = 3136X; \frac{800000}{3136} = X ; 255.1 \text{ mR} = X$$

(See p. 68)

Density Maintenance Formula

$$\frac{\text{mAs}_1}{\text{mAs}_2} = \frac{(SID)^2_1}{(SID)^2_1}$$

For example, optimal density is achieved at an SID of 40 inches using 25 mAs. The SID must be increased to 56 inches. What adjustment in mAs is needed to maintain radiographic density?

$$\frac{25}{\text{mAs}_2} = \frac{(40)^2}{(56)^2}; 1600 \times = 78,400 \; \frac{78,400}{1600} ; \text{mAs}_2 = 49$$

(See p. 69)

Adjusting mAs for Changes in Grid

A quality radiograph is obtained using 2 mAs @ 70 kVp without using a grid. What new mAs is needed when adding a 12:1 grid to maintain radiographic density?

$$\frac{2\ \text{mAs}}{X} = \frac{1}{5}$$

$$2\ \text{mAs} \times 5 = 1\ X;\ 10\ \text{mAs} = X$$

(See p. 71)

Adjusting mAs for changes in Film-Screen System Speed

A quality radiograph is obtained using 25 mAs @ 80 kVp and 100 speed film-screen system. What new mAs is used to maintain radiographic density when changing to a 400 speed film-screen system?

$$\frac{25\ \text{mAs}}{X} = \frac{400\ \text{spd.}}{100\ \text{spd.}}$$

$$25\ \text{mAs} \times 100 = 400X;\ \frac{2500}{400} = 6.25\ \text{mAs} = X$$

(See p. 72)

Adjusting mAs for Changes in Part Thickness

An optimal radiograph was obtained using 40 mAs on an anatomic part that measured 18 cm. The same anatomic part is radiographed in another patient, and it measures 22 cm. What new mAs is needed to maintain density? Because the part thickness was increased by 4 cm, the original mAs is multiplied by 2, yielding 80 mAs. **(See p. 73)**

CHAPTER 5: RADIOGRAPHIC IMAGE QUALITY: GEOMETRIC PROPERTIES

Calculating Geometric Unsharpness

The amount of geometric unsharpness can be calculated for each of the following images to determine which image has greater geometric unsharpness.

Image 1
Focal spot size = 0.6 mm
SID = 40 inches
OID = 0.25 inch

Image 2
Focal spot size = 1.2 mm
SID = 56 inches
OID = 4.0 inches

Image 1
$$\frac{0.6\ \text{mm} \times 0.25\ \text{inch}}{39.75\ \text{inches}};\ \frac{0.15}{39.75}$$

Image 2
$$\frac{1.2\ \text{mm} \times 4\ \text{inches}}{52\ \text{inches}};\ \frac{4.8}{52}$$

Geometric unsharpness of Image 1 = 0.004 mm
Geometric unsharpness of Image 2 = 0.09 mm

Image 2 has the greater amount of unsharpness.

(See p. 108)

The Magnification Factor

A posteroanterior (PA) projection of the chest was produced with an SID of 72 inches and an OID of 3 inches. What is the MF?

$$MF = \frac{72 \text{ inches}}{69 \text{ inches}}$$
$$MF = 1.044$$

(See p. 117)

Determining Object Size

On a PA chest film taken with an SID of 72 inches and an OID of 3 inches (SOD is equal to 69 inches), the size of a round lesion in the right lung measures 1.5 inches in diameter on the radiograph. The MF has been determined to be 1.044. What is the object size of this lesion?

$$\text{Object size} = \frac{1.5 \text{ inches}}{1.044}$$
$$\text{Object size} = 1.44 \text{ inches}$$

(See p. 118)

CHAPTER 6: SCATTER CONTROL

Calculating Grid Ratio

What is the grid ratio when the lead strips are 3.2 mm high and separated by 0.2 mm?

$$\text{Grid ratio} = h/D$$
$$\text{Grid ratio} = \frac{3.2}{0.2}$$
$$= 16 \text{ or } 16:1$$

(See p. 139)

Adding a Grid

If a radiographer produced a knee radiograph with a non-grid exposure using 10 mAs and next wanted to use an 8:1 grid, what mAs should be used to produce a radiograph with the same density?

Nongrid exposure = 10 mAs

GCF (for 8:1 grid) = 4 (from Table 6-2)

$$GCF = \frac{\text{mAs with the grid}}{\text{mAs without the grid}}$$
$$4 = \frac{\text{mAs with the grid}}{10}$$
$$40 = \text{mAs with the grid}$$

When adding an 8:1 grid, the mAs must be increased by a factor of 4, in this case to 40 mAs.

(See p. 145)

Removing a Grid

If a radiographer produced a knee radiograph using a 16:1 grid and 60 mAs, and on the next exposure wanted to use a non-grid exposure, what mAs should be used to produce a radiograph with the same density?

Grid exposure = 60 mAs

GCF (for 16:1 grid) = 6 (from Table 6-2)

$$GCF = \frac{mAs \text{ with the grid}}{mAs \text{ without the grid}}$$

$$6 = \frac{60}{mAs \text{ without the grid}}$$

$$10 = mAs \text{ without the grid}$$

When removing a 16:1 grid, the mAs must be decreased by a factor of 6, in this case to 10 mAs.
(See p. 145)

Increasing the Grid Ratio

If a radiographer performed a routine portable abdomen exam using 30 mAs with a 6:1 grid, what mAs should be used if a 12:1 grid is used?

Exposure 1: 30 mAs, 6:1 grid, GCF = 3

Exposure 2: _____ mAs, 12:1 grid, GCF = 5

$$\frac{mAs_1}{mAs_2} = \frac{GCF_1}{GCF_2}$$

$$\frac{30}{mAs_2} = \frac{3}{5}$$

$$mAs_2 = 50$$

Increasing the grid ratio requires additional mAs.
(See p. 146)

Decreasing the Grid Ratio

If a radiographer used 40 mAs with an 8:1 grid, what mAs should be used with a 5:1 grid in order to produce the same density?

Exposure 1: 40 mAs, 8:1 grid, GCF = 4

Exposure 2: _____ mAs, 5:1 grid, GCF = 2

$$\frac{mAs_1}{mAs_2} = \frac{GCF_1}{GCF_2}$$

$$\frac{40}{mAs_2} = \frac{4}{2}$$

$$mAs_2 = 20$$

Decreasing the grid ratio requires less mAs.
(See p. 146)

CHAPTER 7: IMAGE RECEPTORS

The Intensification Factor

If a radiograph of a hand was produced with 100 mAs using direct exposure and a radiograph of the same hand was produced with an intensifying screen system using 4 mAs, resulting in the same density as the first film, what is the IF of the screen system?

$$IF = \frac{\text{Exposure required without screens}}{\text{Exposure required with screens}}$$

$$IF = \frac{100 \text{ mAs}}{4 \text{ mAs}}$$

$$IF = 25$$

This indicates that 25 times the exposure would be needed to produce a radiograph with comparable density if a direct-exposure system were used. (See p. 175)

Use of the mAs Conversion Formula for Screens

If 10 mAs were used with a 400 speed screen system to produce an optimal radiograph, what mAs would be necessary to produce a radiograph with the same density using a 100 speed screen system?

$$\frac{mAs_1}{mAs_2} = \frac{\text{Relative screen speed}_2}{\text{Relative screen speed}_1}$$

$$\frac{10 \text{ mAs}}{mAs_2} = \frac{100 \text{ relative speed}}{400 \text{ relative speed}}$$

$$mAs_2 = 40$$

When changing from a 400 speed system to a 100 speed system, one needs 4 times the mAs to maintain density. This also means that the patient receives 4 times the radiation dose.
(See p. 176)

CHAPTER 9: SENSITOMETRY

Using Sensitometry to Calculate Exposure Technique Changes

60 mAs produced an image density of 2.05 (log E – 1.54). What mAs would produce an image density of 1.30 (log E = 1.38)?
Subtract log E of the original density (2.05) from the log E of the desired density (1.30):

$$1.38$$
$$\underline{-1.54}$$
$$-0.16; \text{ antilog of } -0.16 = 0.69$$

Multiply the original mAs by 0.69:

$$60 \text{ mAs} \times 0.69 = 41.4 \text{ mAs}$$

Changing the original optical density on the repeat radiograph from 2.05 to 1.30 requires the mAs to be decreased to 41.4. (See p. 238)

Calculating Average Gradient

$$\text{Average gradient} = \frac{D_2 - D_1}{E_2 - E_1}$$

where

$$D_1 = \text{OD } 0.25 + 0.17 \text{ (B + F)}$$
$$D_2 = \text{OD } 2.0 + 0.17 \text{ (B + F)}$$
$$E_1 = \text{Exposure that produces } D_1$$
$$E_2 = \text{Exposure that produces } D_2$$

Example:

$$\frac{2.17 - 0.42}{1.46 - 0.8} = \frac{1.75}{0.66} = 2.65 \text{ Average gradient}$$

(See p. 241)

Summary of Practical Tips

CHAPTER 2: THE X-RAY BEAM

Using the Anode Heel Effect

The anode heel effect can be used in imaging the thoracic spine, which has small vertebrae at the top and large vertebrae at the bottom. By placing the patient's head under the anode end of the tube, the more intense radiation will be directed toward the lower, larger portion of the spine and less intense radiation will expose the upper, smaller vertebrae. (See p. 35)

CHAPTER 3: RADIOGRAPHIC IMAGE FORMATION

X-Ray Interaction with Matter

When the diagnostic primary x-ray beam interacts with anatomic tissues, three processes occur during attenuation of the x-ray beam: absorption, scattering, and transmission. (See p. 50)

CHAPTER 4: RADIOGRAPHIC IMAGE QUALITY: PHOTOGRAPHIC PROPERTIES

Repeating Radiographs Because of Density Errors

The minimum change needed to correct for a density error is determined by multiplying or dividing the mAs by 2. When a greater change in mAs is needed, the radiographer should multiply or divide by 4, 8, and so on. (See p. 63)

Kilovoltage and the 15% Rule

A 15% increase in kilovoltage peak will have the same effect on radiographic density as doubling the mAs. A 15% decrease in kVp will have the same effect on radiographic density as decreasing the mAs by half. (See p. 66)

Altering SID between 40 and 72 Inches

When a 72-inch SID cannot be used, adjusting the SID to 56 inches requires half the mAs. When a 40-inch SID cannot be used, adjusting the SID to 56 inches requires twice the mAs. This quick method of calculating mAs changes should produce sufficient density. (See p. 69)

Selection of Exposure Factors for use with Contrast Media

The radiographer should select a high kVp (90 and above) for barium sulfate studies and a medium kVp (70 to 80) for procedures requiring iodinated solutions. (See p. 86)

CHAPTER 5: RADIOGRAPHIC IMAGE QUALITY: GEOMETRIC PROPERTIES

Selecting Focal Spot Size

The radiographer should select the smallest focal spot size, considering the amount of x-ray exposure used and the amount of recorded detail required for the radiographic examination. (See p. 105)

Minimizing Geometric Unsharpness

The radiographer should select the smallest focal spot size when maximal recorded detail is important; he or she should also consider the amount of heat load within the x-ray tube. In addition, the radiographer should select the standard SID when OID is minimal. When increased OID is unavoidable, SID should be increased slightly to compensate. (See p. 109)

Eliminating Motion

Patient motion can be controlled by the following:

1. Using short exposure times compensated for by higher mA
2. Providing clear instructions for the patient to assist in immobilization
3. Using physical immobilization, such as sandbags, tape, or other devices, as deemed necessary.
   (See p. 113)

Minimizing OID

The radiographer should always try to minimize OID as much as possible to reduce size distortion (magnification). Within the protocol of the examination, it is always best to try to position the area of interest closest to the image receptor to minimize size distortion of that area. (See p. 114)

Minimizing Shape Distortion

Elongation and foreshortening can be minimized by ensuring the proper CR alignment of the following:

1. X-ray tube
2. Part
3. Image receptor
4. Entry or exit point of the CR

(See p. 119)

CHAPTER 6: SCATTER CONTROL

The Role of the Radiographer

In performing radiographic exams, the radiographer both selects the kVp and adjusts the beam restriction. It is up to each radiographer to use the kVp appropriate to the exam and to limit the x-ray beam field size to the anatomic area of interest. (See p. 127)

Compensating for Collimation

When collimating significantly (changing from an 11- × 14-inch field size to a small, 4-inch-diameter cone), the radiographer must increase exposure to compensate for the loss of density that otherwise occurs. The kilovoltage peak (kVp) value should not be increased because it results in decreased contrast. To change density only, mAs should be changed. (See p. 130)

Limit Field Size to Image Receptor Size

The size of the projected radiation field should never exceed the size of the image receptor. This will ensure patient protection from excessive radiation exposure while also improving image quality. (See p. 136)

When to use a grid

A grid should be used when the anatomic part being imaged is 10 cm or more (typically the size of an adult knee) and more than 60 kVp is appropriate for the exam. (See p. 137)

Using upside down focused grid

Upside down focused grid error is easily avoided because every focused grid should have a label indicating "Tube Side." This side of the grid should always face the tube, away from the image receptor. (See p. 148)

Grid Selection

Grids differ from one another in performance, especially in the areas of grid ratio and focal distance. Before using a grid, the radiographer must determine the grid ratio so that the appropriate exposure factors can be selected. Also, the radiographer must be aware of the focal range of focused grids so that the appropriate SID is selected. Box 6-1 lists attributes of the grid typically used in radiography. (See p. 153)

Making the Air Gap Technique Work

Using an increased OID is necessary for the air gap technique. However, this decreases image quality. To decrease unsharpness and increase recorded detail, the radiographer must increase SID. (See p. 154)

Shielding the IR when making more than one exposure

Because digital imaging systems are highly sensitive to low energy radiation, the radiographer should place lead shields over the areas not being exposed when including more than one image on the IR. (See p. 155)

CHAPTER 7: IMAGE RECEPTORS

Spectral Emission and Spectral Sensitivity

The spectral emission of intensifying screens must be matched to the spectral sensitivity of the film. The spectral emission of safelight filters in the darkroom must be compatible with the spectral sensitivity of the film. (See p. 169)

Selecting a Screen Speed

The radiographer should select the film-screen system that balances patient exposure and recorded detail. (See p. 177)

Identifying Cassettes

When it is necessary to find the specific cassette that has a problem, it can be done easily by numbering the cassettes. An excellent way to accomplish this is to write the cassette number (by use of a permanent black marker) in an out-of-the-way corner on the surface of one of the screens. That same number should be written on the outside of the cassette. The screen number will show up on images produced with that cassette, and if there is a problem, knowledge of this number allows the radiographer to find and test the cassette in question. (See p. 182)

Erasure of Imaging Plates

If CR imaging plates are not used within 48 hours, they should be put through an erasure cycle before use. (See p. 185)

Avoiding Fading of Latent Image

CR imaging plates should be processed within 1 hour of exposure; otherwise, fading of the latent image will begin to impact image quality. (See p. 185)

Adjusting the mAs for CR

When using CR, it is appropriate to adjust the mAs as if using a 200 speed film-screen system. Since many regular film-screen combinations are 400 speed, this requires doubling the mAs. (See p. 185)

CHAPTER 8: RADIOGRAPHIC FILM PROCESSING

Film Orientation for Proper Replenishment

The radiographer should align the radiographic film so that the film is horizontally placed on the feed tray and its leading edge is long. When processing two 8 × 10-inch films, the radiographer should place both films parallel to each other so that the leading edges are short. (See p. 206)

CHAPTER 9: SENSITOMETRY

Sensitometric Curves Position along the X Axis

Sensitometric curves of faster-speed film are positioned to the left of slower-speed film, and sensitometric curves of slower-speed film are positioned to the right of faster-speed film. (See p. 236)

Changes in Exposure Technique to Correct for Density Errors

To correct for the density error, optical densities that lie outside the straight-line region of the sensitometric curve (toe or shoulder region) require a greater or lesser change in exposure than those that lie within the straight-line region. (See p. 245)

Achieving Maximum Film Contrast

To achieve the maximum contrast that the film is capable of producing, the radiographer must ensure that the optical densities lie within the straight-line region of the sensitometric curve. (See p. 245)

CHAPTER 10: EXPOSURE FACTOR SELECTION

Technique Chart Limitations

Exposure technique charts are designed for the typical or average patient. Patient variability in terms of body build or physical condition, or the presence of a pathologic condition, requires the radiographer to solve problems when selecting exposure factors. (See p. 253)

Equipment Performance

Radiography equipment must be operating within normal limits for technique charts to be effective. (See p. 254)

Measurement of Part Thickness

Accurate measurement of part thickness is critical to the effective use of exposure technique charts. (See p. 254)

Applicability of a Variable kVp/Fixed mAs Technique Chart

Variable kVp technique charts may be more effective when small extremities are being imaged. (See p. 257)

Fixed kVp/Variable mAs and Part Measurement

Accuracy of measurement is less critical with fixed kVp/variable mAs technique charts than with variable kVp/fixed mAs technique charts. (See p. 259)

CHAPTER 11: AUTOMATIC EXPOSURE CONTROL

AEC, kVp, and Radiographic Contrast

Assuming the radiographer is selecting or using a kVp value above the minimum needed to penetrate the part, adjustment of this value does not affect density when an AEC device is used. It does affect radiographic contrast, however (Figure 11-7). The radiographer must be sure to set the kVp value as needed to ensure adequate penetration and to produce the appropriate scale of contrast. (See p. 274)

AEC and Density Settings

Routinely using plus or minus density settings to produce acceptable radiographs indicates that a problem exists, possibly a problem with the AEC device. (See p. 275)

AEC and Non-Bucky Studies

The radiographer should be certain to deactivate the AEC system and use a manual technique when performing any radiographic study where the image receptor is located outside of the Bucky. (See p. 277)

AEC and mAs Readout

If the radiographic unit has a mAs readout display, the radiographer should be sure to notice the reading after the exposure is made. This information can be invaluable. (See p. 278)

AEC Calibration and Computed Radiography (CR)

As indicated in Chapter 7, the sensitivity of CR systems is approximately equivalent to a 200 speed film-screen system. In order to achieve optimal digital image quality, AEC devices used with CR image receptors should be recalibrated to ensure that the exposure to the IP is correct. (See p. 281)

CHAPTER 12: DIGITAL IMAGING

Exposure Technique Selection and Digital Imaging

Optimal exposure techniques should be selected regardless of whether film-screen or digital image receptors are used. Although the digital imaging system can adjust for exposure technique errors, poor image quality or increased radiation exposure to the patient may result. (See p. 308)

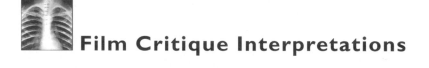

Film Critique Interpretations

CHAPTER 4: RADIOGRAPHIC IMAGE QUALITY: PHOTOGRAPHIC PROPERTIES

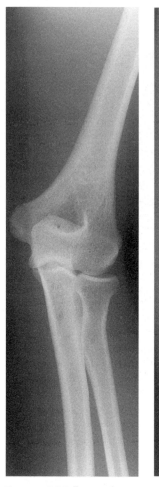

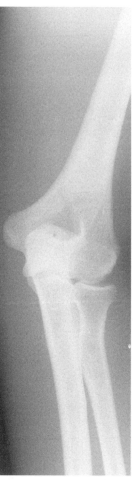

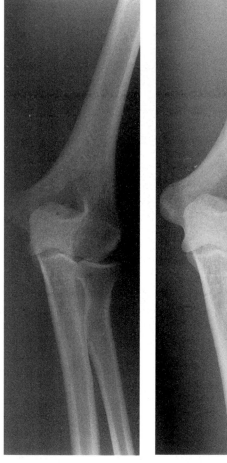

FIGURE 4-26 Image A was produced using 60 kVp, 100 mA at 0.040 s, 100 speed film-screen combination, 40-inch SID, and minimal OID.

FIGURE 4-27 Image B was produced using 60 kVp, 80 mA at 0.025 s, 100 speed film-screen combination, 40-inch SID, and minimal OID.

FIGURE 4-28 Image C was produced using 69 kVp, 160 mA at 0.025 s, 100 speed film-screen combination, 40-inch SID, and minimal OID.

FIGURE 4-29 Image D was produced using 60 kVp, 200 mA at 0.020 s, 100 speed film-screen combination, 40-inch SID, and 3-inch OID.

1. Given Image A is of optimal quality, discuss the quality of the other images.

   Image B The radiographic density of this image is insufficient (too light) to visualize all of the anatomic structures. Radiographic contrast and recorded detail cannot be evaluated because the image is too light.

   Image C The radiographic density of this image is excessive (too dark) to adequately visualize all of the anatomic structures. Radiographic contrast and recorded detail cannot be evaluated because the image is too dark.

   Image D The radiographic density of this image is slightly lower than that of Image A. Radiographic contrast appears slightly higher than that of Image A. Differences in recorded detail are difficult to visualize, but the image appears magnified in comparison to Image A.

2. For each image, evaluate its exposure variables and discuss their effect on the quality of the image, regardless of whether it is apparent on the radiograph.

   Image B The kVp is the same as that used in Image A; therefore the radiographic contrast would be equal. The mAs used is 2, demonstrating a change in the intensity of exposure from Image A by half which results in less radiographic density. All other exposure factors remain the same, producing the same amount of recorded detail as in Image A.

   Image C The kVp is 15% higher than the kVp used in Image A. This increases the intensity of exposure by a factor of 2 and results in greater radiographic density. The mAs used (4) is the same as used in Image A. All other exposure factors are equal, so the amount of recorded detail is equal to that of Image A.

   Image D The kVp and mAs are the same as those used in Image A. The only exposure factor changed is the object-to-image receptor distance (OID). An increase in OID (3 inches) increases the size of the image (magnification) and results in less scatter radiation reaching the film. This increases the radiographic contrast and decreases radiographic density.

3. For each image, identify any adjustments that could be made in the exposure factors to produce an image comparable to Image A.

   Image B To increase the radiographic density, the radiographer must increase the mAs by a factor of 2. The mA can be doubled (160 mA at 0.025 = 4 mAs), or the time of exposure can be doubled (80 mA at 0.050 = 4 mAs).

   Image C To decrease the radiographic density, the radiographer must decrease the mAs by a factor of 2 or decrease the kVp by 15%. A kVp of 69 produces lower radiographic contrast than a kVp of 60. Therefore changing the kVp to 60 (a 15% decrease) decreases the radiographic density and produces an image comparable to Image A.

   Image D Maintaining the same exposure factors and decreasing the OID to its minimum produces an image comparable to Image A. Decreasing the OID produces an image with less magnification and adds slightly more density because more scatter radiation reaches the film.

CHAPTER 5: RADIOGRAPHIC IMAGE QUALITY: GEOMETRIC PROPERTIES

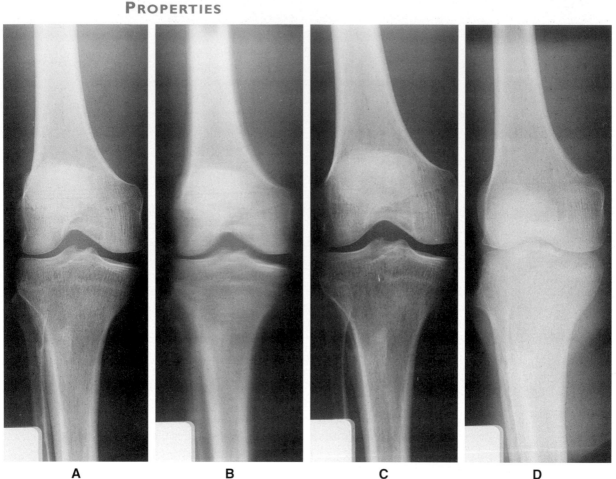

A

B

C

D

FIGURE 5-16 Image **A** was produced using 65 kVp, 100 mA at 0.10 s, 400 speed film-screen combination, 40-inch SID, central ray perpendicular, small focal spot size, and minimal OID.

FIGURE 5-17 Image **B** was produced using 65 kVp, 10 mA at 1.0 s. 400 speed film-screen combination, 40-inch SID, central ray perpendicular, small focal spot size, and minimal OID.

FIGURE 5-18 Image **C** was produced using 65 kVp, 500 mA at 0.20 s, 400 speed film-screen combination, 35-inch SID, central ray perpendicular, large focal spot size, and 2-inch OID.

FIGURE 5-19 Image **D** was produced using 65 kVp, 100 mA at 0.064 s, 600 speed film-screen combination, 44-inch SID, central ray angled 40 degrees caudad, small focal spot size, and minimal OID.

1. Given that Image A is of optimal quality, discuss the quality of the other images.

   Image B The radiographic density and contrast appear sufficient to visualize the anatomic structures and are comparable to Image A. Motion is visible on the image and as a result, recorded detail is decreased, which increases the amount of unsharpness recorded.

   Image C The radiographic density is slightly darker than Image A, but it is acceptable. Radiographic contrast appears appropriate and comparable to Image A. The size of the image appears larger that Image A and results in increased magnification compared to Image A. Increased distortion also results in decreased recorded detail, which increases the amount of unsharpness recorded.

   Image D The radiographic density is insufficient (too light) to visualize all the anatomic structures, and is considerably less than Image A. The radiographic contrast cannot be evaluated because the image is too light. The shape of the anatomic part appears distorted. The knee joint is not open and the patella and fibula are not aligned properly to the tibia and femur as in Image A. The recorded detail is decreased because of shape distortion.

2. For each image, evaluate its exposure variables and discuss their effect on the quality of the image, regardless of whether it is apparent on the radiograph.

   Image B The same kVp and mAs are used and therefore the radiographic density and contrast are sufficient and comparable to Image A. The exposure time is significantly increased from 0.10 s in Image A to 1.0 s in Image B. The increase in exposure time results in motion of the anatomic part. Motion causes the recorded detail to decrease and therefore increases the amount of unsharpness.

   Image C Although the same kVp and mAs are used, the decrease in SID from 40" in Image A to 35" in Image B results in an increase in radiographic density, an increase in magnification, and a decrease in recorded detail. Using the Large Focal Spot increases the amount of unsharpness recorded compared with using the Small Focal Spot in Image A. The increase in OID also contributes to increasing the size of the image and decreasing the amount of recorded detail resulting in increased sharpness. The 2-inch increase in OID has less of an effect on radiographic density than decreasing the SID by 5 inches.

   Image D The same kVp is used but the mAs is decreased from 10 in Image A to 6.4 in Image B. This decrease in mAs appropriately compensates for the increase in the film-screen speed in Image B. The 40-degree angle on the central ray, without a compensating decrease in SID, results in increased SID, and distorts the shape of the anatomic part. The 4-inch increase in SID in Image B results in an increase in the recorded detail, less magnification compared to Image A, and less radiographic density. Although an increase in the SID would typically increase recorded detail and decrease magnification, the distortion of the anatomic part has a greater overall affect on the image.

3. For each image, identify any adjustments that could be made in the exposure factors to produce an image comparable to Image A.

Image B   The exposure time should be decreased and the mA increased proportionally to reduce the possibility of motion of the anatomic part. For example, to obtain a mAs of 10, the exposure time could be decreased to 0.2 s and the mA increased to 50.

Image C   The SID should be increased to 40 inches and the OID reduced as much as possible. Increasing the SID and decreasing the OID improves recorded detail and is comparable to Image A. In addition, the Small Focal Spot should be used to reduce the amount of unsharpness recorded.

Image D   The SID should be reduced to 40 inches and the central ray should be perpendicular to the area of interest. Using a perpendicular central ray reduces the amount of shape distortion and the resulting image is comparable to Image A.

CHAPTER 6: SCATTER CONTROL

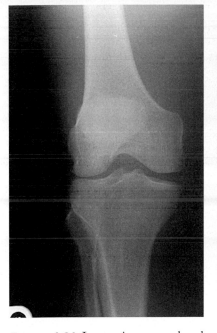 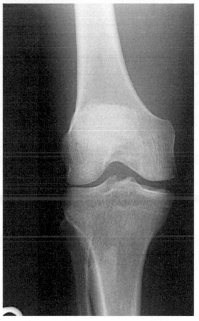

FIGURE 6-26 Image A was produced using 70 kVp, 100 mA at 0.016 s, 400 speed film-screen combination, a 40-inch source-to-image receptor distance, and no grid.

FIGURE 6-27 Image B was produced using 70 kVp, 50 mA at 0.160 s, 400 speed film-screen combination, a 40-inch source-to-image receptor distance, and a 12:1 grid ratio.

1. Evaluate each radiograph and discuss its quality.

   Image A The radiographic density is sufficient to visualize the anatomic structures. Radiographic contrast appears low, decreasing the visibility of recorded detail. The recorded detail is difficult to evaluate, but unsharpness appears minimal.

   Image B The radiographic density is sufficient to visualize the anatomic structures. The radiographic contrast appears high, and visibility of recorded detail is improved compared with that of Image A. The recorded detail is difficult to evaluate, but unsharpness appears minimal.

2. For each image, evaluate its exposure variables and discuss their effect on the quality of the image, regardless of whether it is apparent on the radiograph.

   Image A This image is produced using a nongrid exposure technique. A nongrid exposure technique on an adult knee produces an image with lower radiographic contrast because more scatter radiation reaches the film. The kVp used (70) is the same as that used in Image B. The mAs is less to compensate for the nongrid exposure. The density and recorded detail should be similar to those of Image B.

Image B This image is produced using a 12:1 grid ratio. The result is a higher-contrast image because less scatter radiation reaches the film. The mAs is increased to compensate for the use of a grid. The density and recorded detail should be similar to those of Image A.

3. For each image, identify any adjustments that could be made in the exposure factors to produce an optimal image.

Image A To increase the radiographic contrast and improve the quality of the image, the radiographer can add a 12:1 grid. The mAs should be increased by a factor of 5 to compensate for adding the grid. The new mAs would be 8.

Image B No adjustments are necessary to improve the quality of this image.

CHAPTER 7: IMAGE RECEPTORS

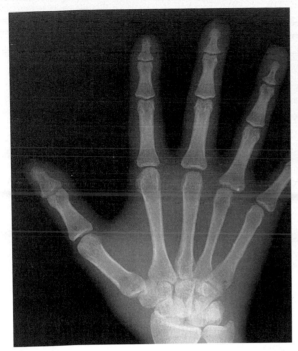 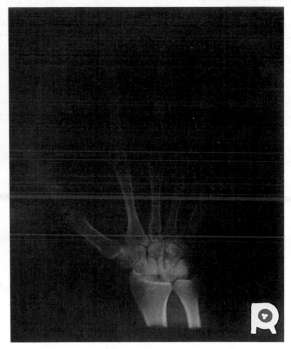

FIGURE 7-18 Image **A** was produced using 57 kVp, 50 mA at 0.040 s, 100 speed film-screen combination, and a 40-inch source-to-image receptor distance.

FIGURE 7-19 Image **B** was produced using 57 kVp, 160 mA at 0.0125 s, 400 speed film-screen combination, and a 40-inch source-to-image receptor distance.

1. Evaluate each radiograph and discuss its quality.
   Image A The radiographic density is sufficient to visualize the anatomic structures. The radiographic contrast is appropriate to visualize the recorded detail. The recorded detail is difficult to evaluate, but unsharpness appears minimal.
   Image B The radiographic density is excessive (too dark), thereby decreasing the visualization of the anatomic structures. The radiographic contrast and recorded detail cannot be evaluated.
2. For each image, evaluate its exposure variables and discuss their effect on the quality of the image, regardless of whether it is apparent on the radiograph.
   Image A The kVp (57) used is appropriate for the level of contrast desired for an extremity radiograph. The mAs (2) used produced sufficient density to visualize the anatomic structures. A 100 film-screen speed combination is appropriate to provide maximum recorded detail.
   Image B The kVp (57) used is appropriate for the level of contrast desired for an extremity radiograph. The mAs (2) used is appropriate for a slower film-screen speed combination. The 400 speed film-screen combination used

produces an image with significantly more density compared with that of Image A. In addition, the recorded detail is lower because of the higher screen speed.

3. For each image, identify any adjustments that could be made in the exposure factors to produce an optimal image.

Image A No adjustments need to be made to improve the quality of this image.

Image B The kVp and mAs are adequate for producing a quality image of the hand. The 400 speed film-screen combination should be changed to a 100 speed film-screen combination. This decreases the radiographic density appropriately. In the event that a lower speed film-screen combination cannot be used, the mAs should be decreased by a factor of 4 to decrease the radiographic density. The new mAs used with the 400 speed film-screen combination would be 0.5.

CHAPTER 11: AUTOMATIC EXPOSURE CONTROL

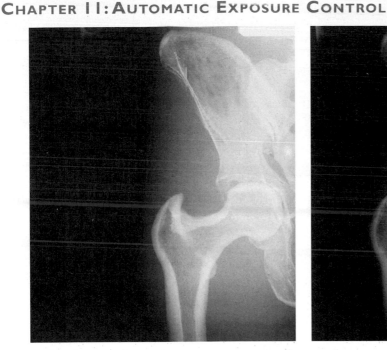

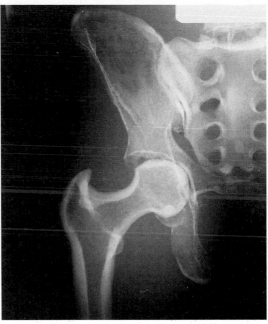

FIGURE 11-9 Image A is produced using 70 kVp, 200 mA, AEC exposure, center detector, 400 speed film-screen combination, and a 40-inch source to-image receptor distance.

FIGURE 11-10 Image B is produced using 70 kVp, 200 mA, AEC exposure, center detector, 400 speed film-screen combination, and a 40-inch source-to-image receptor distance.

1. Evaluate each radiograph and discuss its quality.

   Image A The radiographic density is low, thereby reducing the visibility of some anatomic structures. The radiographic contrast appears appropriate for the anatomic structure. The recorded detail is difficult to evaluate, but unsharpness appears minimal. The central ray centering appears more lateral compared with the positioning used in Image B.

   Image B The radiographic density is sufficient to visualize the anatomic structure. The radiographic contrast is appropriate to visualize the recorded detail. The recorded detail is difficult to evaluate, but unsharpness appears minimal. The central ray centering appears more medial compared with the positioning used in Image A.

2. For each image, evaluate its exposure variables and discuss their effect on the quality of the image (regardless of whether it is apparent on the radiograph).

   Image A The kVp is appropriate for the anatomic structure. The film-screen combination and AEC center detector are appropriate for the hip. The exposure factors are the same as those used in Image B. Although image quality is not equal, exposure factors appear appropriate for the examination.

Image B The kVp is appropriate for the anatomic structure. The film-screen combination and AEC center detector are appropriate for the hip. The exposure factors are the same as those used in Image A. Although image quality is not equal, exposure factors appear appropriate for the examination.

3. For each image, identify any adjustments that could be made in the exposure factors to produce an optimal image.

Image A Given an AEC exposure and the same factors used in Image B, the centering of the central ray should be directed more medially and centered closer to the femoral neck. Improper centering of the central ray produces an image with less density because the hip is not placed correctly over the center detector.

Image B No adjustments need to be made to improve the quality of this image.

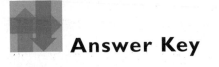

Answer Key

Chapter 1: Radiation and Its Discovery

1. B	2. C	3. D	4. A	5. D
6. C	7. B	8. D	9. A	10. C

Chapter 2: Production of X-Rays

1. B	2. D	3. B	4. A	5. C
6. A	7. D	8. A	9. C	10. D
11. D	12. B			

Chapter 3: Radiographic Image Formation

1. D	2. D	3. C	4. B	5. D
6. B	7. A	8. C	9. C	10. A

Chapter 4: Radiographic Image Quality: Photographic Properties

1. B	2. D	3. C	4. D	5. A
6. B	7. B	8. B	9. A	10. C
11. B	12. C	13. B	14. D	15. D

Chapter 5: Radiographic Image Quality: Geometric Properties

1. A	2. C	3. D	4. D	5. B
6. B	7. C	8. D	9. A	10. C

Chapter 6: Scatter Control

1. C	2. B	3. D	4. B	5. B
6. A	7. D	8. D	9. B	10. A
11. D	12. A	13. C	14. C	15. A
16. B	17. C	18. D		

Chapter 7: Image Receptors

1. B	2. C	3. A	4. B	5. C
6. C	7. C	8. D	9. B	10. D
11. B	12. C	13. A	14. C	15. D
16. D	17. A	18. D	19. A	20. C

Chapter 8: Radiographic Film Processing

1. B	2. C	3. C	4. A	5. D
6. C	7. B	8. C	9. D	10. A
11. C	12. D	13. C	14. B	15. A

Chapter 9: Sensitometry

1. D	2. C	3. D	4. B	5. A
6. C	7. B	8. A	9. A	10. C

Chapter 10: Exposure Factor Selection

1. C	2. B	3. C	4. A	5. D
6. B	7. C	8. B	9. D	10. A

Chapter 11: Automatic Exposure Control

1. C	2. B	3. C	4. D	5. D
6. B	7. D	8. B	9. A	10. C
11. C	12. E			

Chapter 12: Digital Imaging

1. B	2. D	3. B	4. D	5. B
6. C	7. C	8. C	9. A	10. B
11. D	12. B			

Fluoroscopy
  characteristics of, 52-54, 53f
  digital, 54, 296
Focal distance, 142
Focal range, 142, 143f
Focal spot, 17-18
  size of, 32-33, 34f, 103-105, 103f, 104f
Focused grid, 140, 141f, 142
Focusing cup, 15
Focusing lens, electrostatic, 52-53
Fog
  chemical, 197
  definition of, 51
Foreign object as artifact, 221f
Foreshortening, 118, 119f
Formula
  for adding or removing grid, 145
  for average gradient, 241
  density maintenance, 68
  film speed, 237-238, 238b, 238f
  geometric unsharpness, 108, 108b
  grid ratio, 139, 146
  inverse square law, 68
  optical density, 230b
Frequency
  grid, 138
  wavelength and, 6-9, 8f
Front screen, 173

G

Gamma, 241
Generator output, 74
Geometric property, 102, 102f
Geometric unsharpness, 103-109
  distance and, 105-109, 105f-107f
  focal spot size and, 103-105, 103f, 104f
Glass envelope, 18
Gradient, average, 240-241, 240f
Gradient point, 239
Grid, 136-153
  adding or removing, 145
  construction of, 138-139, 138f
  contrast and, 81
  cutoff errors of, 147-152, 148f-151f
  density and, 70-71
  focused or non-focused, 140, 141f-143f, 142-143
  pattern of, 139-140, 140f
  performance of, 144-147, 144t
  selection of, 153
  stationary and reciprocating, 143
  when to use, 137, 152-153
Grid conversion factor, 144, 144t
Grid frequency, 138

Grid ratio, 138
  density and, 144
  dose and, 146
  increasing or decreasing, 146
Guide plate, 202, 204f

H

Half-value layer, 36
Hardener, 197, 198
Hazard to film, 215
Health Level Seven standard, 315
Heat, dissipating, 17
Heat unit, 38-39
Heater, immersion, 210
High-contrast image, 77, 77f
Histogram, 301-302
Housing, x-ray tube, 18-19, 18f, 19f
Hypersthenic body habitus, 90f, 91-92
Hyposthenic body habitus, 90, 90f

I

Image
  digital. *See* Digital imaging
  formation of, 45-55
    absorption and, 47-48, 48f
    beam attenuation and, 47-55
    differential absorption and, 46-47, 46f
    exit radiation and, 51-54, 51f-53f
    scattering and, 48-50, 49f
    transmission and, 50, 50f
  latent. *See* Latent image
  manifest, 164, 194
  postprocessing enhancement of, 293, 304, 305f-307f, 308
  quality of
    contrast and, 76-87. *See also* Contrast
    density affecting, 55-76. *See also* Density
    exposure and, 87-97. *See also* Exposure
    sharpness and, 102-124. *See also* Sharpness
    visibility and, 54, 55f
Image intensification, 52
Image receptor, 46, 160-189
  cassette for, 183, 184f
  computed radiography, 184-185
  digital, 183-184, 185f, 292, 292f
  direct readout digital, 185, 186f
  film as, 162-170. *See also* Film
  film-screen, 302f
  intensifying screen as, 171-182. *See also* Intensifying screen
  scatter and, 126, 155
Image receptor contrast, 77
Image receptor unsharpness, 109-111, 110f
Imaging plate, 184, 185f, 297
Immersion heater, 210, 211f
Indirect conversion detector, 300-301